Naturally
Healthy at Home

Holistic solutions for the
improved well-being of yourself,
friends and family.

by
Dr. Valeria Breiten

Naturally Healthy at Home

INTRODUCTION

    This book is intended as a guide for home health care, helping anyone who would like to have a different kind of home medicine chest. My focus is on safe therapies that support the body in healing itself. Mothers of young children have especially appreciated this information in dealing with falls and tumbles. It is similar having a knowledgeable grandmother on hand.

    The table of contents list the major topics that are covered, in an easily accessible and understandable format. A shopping list is in the appendix of supplies to have on hand, especially for sudden onset problems.

Best wishes,

Dr. Valeria Breiten
Ashland, Oregon

Contents

ALLERGIES AND ASTHMA

Allergies are symptoms of an immune system overreacting to items such as dust, molds, pollens or foods. Asthma and eczema are generally allergic reactions that are chronic.

HAY FEVER

Hay fever season can occur at different times of the year, depending on what pollen causes an allergic reaction and when that tree or flower pollinates. Many people have problems in the spring or fall with hay fever. The best treatment is to go to your homeopath during the season for an acute remedy to help the immediate symptoms, and then again at the end of your hay fever season to have a constitutional remedy prescribed. A constitutional homeopathic remedy will help your body's immune system re-calibrate so that it will stop overreacting. Healing can be a gradual process. Every year the allergy symptoms are better. For individuals with mild hay fever, it may clear and not return. For others that have done many different therapies over many years, it can be a process of healing and improving every year.

While your body is healing, here are some tips on how to deal with the discomfort of the season. A saltwater nasal wash is easy and very effective. My friend, Ric, was surprised how successful and easy it was. His first reaction to snorting saltwater was not optimistic! But it really worked well. Buy a Neti pot at your local health food store. The intention is to have the saltwater go into one nostril with your head tilted, then drain out the other nostril. The saltwater is a mixture of ½ teaspoon salt to ½ cup of water. It washes out the pollen that is irritating inside the nostrils and relief is very quick. I recommend using it before bedtime or after being outside and exposed to allergens, but it is safe to use as many times as needed throughout the day.

Itchy eyes can also be very distressing. Washing the eyes with cool water and an under the tongue dose of homeopathic Pulsatilla 30C frequently relieves the itching, especially if the condition is accompanied by a bland yellow discharge and feeling weepy.

The most successful item I've found for opening the nose and sinuses for sleeping is a lavender steam just before bedtime. To do an herbal steam, place a tablespoon of the herb in a large mixing bowl and add two cups of boiling water. Place it on a table and sit with a towel over your head, your nose over the bowl and breathe the steam coming from the tea.

Nasal strips, a special strip you can buy that goes over the top of the nose, can help improve the airflow, particularly at night, by gently pulling open the nasal passages. Staying hydrated by drinking plenty of water or herbal teas during the day and using a humidifier plus air purifier, especially in your sleeping area at night, will help keep things flowing. The essential oil of Marjoram or Thyme applied under the nose is helpful to increase air flow while sleeping.

You can reduce runny noses and congestion from allergies with freeze-dried nettles capsules taken three times a day. The herb has a mild drying effect and reduces hay fever symptoms for many people. Nettles are also very mineral dense, so there is a tremendous amount of nutritional support with them.

FOOD SENSITIVITIES

Everyone recognizes the food allergy where hives break out immediately upon eating the offending food or handling the cat. These immediate responses are caused by the immune system activating an IgE or IgA antibody allergic response. However, it is more subtle to recognize the food allergy reactions twenty-four to forty-eight hours after eating the allergic food. This delay can occur with foods that the immune system activates via IgG antibodies. These food allergy symptoms include fatigue, edema, blood sugar spikes, joint pain, stomach upsets, skin rashes and breathing problems. Some of the most common food allergies are dairy products, wheat, soy, fish and shellfish, nuts, eggs and citrus. To determine if you have an unknown food allergy you have two choices – elimination diet or testing.

An elimination diet is avoiding all highly allergenic foods and foods which you know don't agree with you. Keep a diary of everything you eat and when any allergic reactions occur. Writing down everything can help in finding a pattern, especially for delayed reactions like the IgG gives. Read food labels carefully. Federal labeling laws make it easier to know if key allergens are in a food.

When you are symptom-free for several weeks, then it is time to challenge your system with one eliminated food at a time. Decide which food to start with, try it and then observe for two days to see if it causes a reaction. If it does cause a reaction to continue, avoid it and move onto the next item you would like to reintroduce to your diet.

Another way to determine food allergies is a blood test. Frequently IgG food allergy testing is necessary to identify the offending foods because of the delayed, chronic effects. The tests are only available through special laboratories by physician prescription. After avoiding the foods identified on the test results for a month most people are symptom free.

It is important to avoid your allergic foods during treatment with acupuncture or constitutional homeopathy. Treatment will help the body heal and hopefully you will be able to return to problematic foods occasionally but not every day.

There are three easy herbal treatments to do at home. First; add a clove of garlic a day to the diet. Secondly; take Calendula tincture (20 drops added to a glass of water) to assist in the healing of the mucous membranes of the gut irritated by the allergy. Third; the amino acid L-Glutamine, a 500 mg capsule daily, taken at a different time from protein foods, assists the intestines in healing.

ASTHMA

Asthma has increased alarmingly in recent years, both in numbers and severity. In most people it is an allergy problem, an example of an immune system functioning incorrectly. It is important to remember that it can be a dangerous and even fatal disease. If you have asthma you cannot rely only on home remedies. You must discuss with a health provider how you can monitor your asthma at home and when you should seek medical attention.

A neighbor of mine was distraught to be told by her doctor that she had to move out of the valley because she had such terrible asthma. She came to see me, and we developed a diet plan for avoiding her food allergies. I also prescribed a classical homeopathic medicine that fit her symptoms and personality plus herbal medicines. She improved so much that not only was she able to stay in town, she was able to stop all of her asthma medicines (with the prescribing physician's approval)!

Asthma is characterized by wheezing and breathlessness from spasms of the bronchi. It is also closely associated with psoriasis and eczema. Learning what your allergic triggers are is very important. Frequently food allergies contribute to the severity of the reaction. Drinking plenty of water and expectorant herb teas such as lavender, chamomile or licorice will help to keep the mucous moving. An herbal tincture of Hawthorne can be helpful, when taken daily as a preventative and a dropperful at the first sign of wheezing.

Sometimes a chamomile or lavender steam at the first sign of problems will help keep the chest loose. To do an herbal steam, place a tablespoon of the herb in a bowl and add two cups of boiling water. Place it on a table and sit with a towel over your head and the bowl so you breathe the steam coming from the tea.

Yoga breathing exercises can help to keep the airways more comfortable. Keeping the mouth closed during inhalation can be very helpful in regulating breathing. In addition, you can breathe out to a count of eight, then hold four counts, breathe in to a count of eight, then hold four counts. Do this repeatedly, in a circular fashion, starting at whatever numbers you can do and working up as your breathing improves. This breathing exercise will both calm you and help your body.

Reduce allergy reactions by creating a safe place to sleep. This is especially important for people with symptoms worse at night or in the morning. Thoroughly clean and remove any possible allergens in the bed and the bedroom. Have washable bed covers and pillows and wash them weekly. Remove the carpet and drapes and replace them with wood floors and blinds and use a Hepa filter vaccum to clean them weekly. Have pets sleep and live away from the bedroom. Be aware of mold in the house and treat it promptly.

Run an air purifier every night in the room while you are sleeping. These changes will keep dust, pollen and dander out of the air you breathe while you are sleeping. When you improve your sleep then general health improves too.

GLUTEN FREE

Recently, a patient, Sara, told me she was eating some gluten-free products she had bought, but wondered what gluten was. I had to chuckle to myself, because she had caught on to the new craze of products available but didn't understand the reason for them. I explained to her that gluten-free is essential for people with Celiac Disease. It is now thought that one out of every one hundred people in the United States has the genes for celiac disease, the disease that is basically a wheat family allergy. This has made the gluten free foods market a huge growth area and you can see foods labeled gluten free in many places.

Celiac disease is a genetically inherited condition that results in inflammation and bleeding of the small intestines. It may not be apparent during much of a person's life, but stresses can trigger it unexpectedly. Some children have immediate symptoms of irritability, diarrhea and failure to grow. Adults might show symptoms of diarrhea, constipation, anemia and osteoporosis. But these symptoms could also be due to an autoimmune disease like Hashimoto's, Rheumatoid Arthritis, Lupus or Diabetes. The patient may come in with Chronic Fatigue Syndrome, muscle aches or joint aches. I have seen mental problems like Attention Disorders, Depression and Bi-polar Disorder respond positively to a gluten-free diet. If one person in the family has been diagnosed with Celiac Disease, then all the relatives should suspect it for themselves and be tested.

The celiac gluten is in only one botanical family, the one with wheat in it. That family includes wheat, rye, spelt, barley, kamut and triticale and all have to be scrupulously avoided. It used to be thought that oats were also a problem, but they are grown and milled with wheat and so it is frequently a contamination issue and gluten-free oats can be purchased. This means the small amounts of wheat in soy sauce to the large amounts in most baked goods, breads and pastas all must be avoided. Eating something that was prepared on the same surface or in the same machine as a wheat product can cause a reaction in sensitive individuals. Even very small amounts can keep the inflammation fully activated, but the reaction may not be immediate – many people experience their reactions several hours and up to 48 hours later which can be confusing especially if, like most people, they eat wheat products many times a day.

There are three main ways to establish a diagnosis of Celiac Disease. A biopsy of the small intestines can be taken and checked for the distinctive tissue changes celiac causes. The biopsy is considered the gold standard for diagnosis by the conventional medical community, but it is invasive and not reliable if cortisone has been taken. The second way is to have blood tests for an allergy to gluten – called anti-gliadin antibodies. This test is expensive if you are not insured and is about 90% reliable. If you have been avoiding gluten, the antibodies could be too low to test in the blood. The third way is to eliminate gluten completely from the diet for 30 days and then do a challenge by eating it three times in one day. Next wait for two days to see if there is a reaction. This only works well if the gluten is totally eliminated before the reintroduction. It can also serve as the beginning of treatment. Genetic testing can also be done, but it doesn't show the difference between the possibility of the disease and actually having it.

The good news about Celiac Disease is that when a person with Celiac completely eliminates gluten from their diet, some amazing healing can occur. In addition to the gluten-free diet, I recommend at least a year of high potency vitamin and mineral supplementation to make up for the malnourishment that occurs when the intestines are chronically inflamed. The minerals seem to be especially affected and are very important to replace in an easily absorbable way. Eating a diet with high levels of fiber can be challenging – so eating lots of vegetables and fruits, and high fiber grains like brown rice, millet and quinoa is helpful. Many people also must eliminate other allergens, like dairy products to have good results. The leaky gut that can occur when the intestines are inflamed can produce a variety of other allergies. Completely eliminating gluten so the intestines can heal often clears the many other allergies a person has, so those foods can eventually be reintroduced to the diet.

DIGESTIVE UPSETS

GERD

It is ironic that many people who come to see me about acid reflux are on antacids or proton pump inhibitors to try and reduce their stomach acid. Research is showing that these are not good medicines for long-term health and can increase the risk of cardiovascular disease. In addition, the problem frequently is not enough stomach acid. With low acid, food moves through slowly and the upper stomach valve to the esophagus doesn't close properly. The symptoms of heartburn are frequently a result of low stomach acid, rather than too much. The body must be reasonably healthy to produce adequate stomach acid, so it is not unusual for problems to develop as we age or develop with other health issues.

Acid reflux pain comes from the stomach contents rising into the esophagus where they do not belong. This is a result of the stomach valve at the top of the stomach not closing properly. Lying down or bending at the middle will put pressure on the stomach and acid can travel back up the esophagus. Most people are worse lying down, especially right after a meal because then gravity allows the acid to go into the esophagus. The constant burning and inflammation can create significant health problems in the esophagus, so it needs to be treated effectively.

Natural treatments include placing wood blocks or bricks under the head of the bed to raise it 4 to 6 inches, so you are sleeping at an angle. It does not work to use more pillows, or sleep in a recliner, because that increases the pressure on the stomach area when you fold in the middle. You want to be able to lie flat, but with your head higher than your feet. For some people this is all it takes to resolve their reflux pain.

My herbal medicine recommendation is to take Ginger and Gentiana, 2 capsules or 20 drops of tincture, before each meal. This helps the food move through faster and seems to help the valve close better, so there is no longer the reflux problem. I don't recommend Peppermint for reflux because it can increase the relaxation of the valve at the top of the stomach.

A sublingual (under the tongue) vitamin B12, dissolved under the tongue daily, is important for people with GERD. B12 won't directly help the reflux problem, rather it treats the other symptoms that can occur because of B12's poor absorption when there are stomach acid problems. B12 requires intrinsic factor made in the stomach to be absorbed in the intestines. The sublingual form of B12 bypasses all of this by going through the mouth membrane directly into the blood stream. B12 shots also bypass the digestion issues.   B12 is important for the well being of the bones and the nerves.

A doctor trained in visceral manipulation can also help the stomach reposition itself so the valve works better, eliminating reflux symptoms.

INDIGESTION

Ginger capsules can be convenient and helpful in moving the digestion along. Many people are helped with two ginger capsules when they realize their digestion is feeling heavy. I have found that if I have indigestion and take two ginger capsules, then take two more if I have no relief within thirty minutes, the problem clears. If indigestion, gas or reflux is interfering with sleep or is happening regularly, then see a physician to assess the cause.

Ginger capsules, tincture or crystallized ginger can be helpful for a variety of stomach upsets including motion sickness or morning sickness. It generally settles the stomach and prevents vomiting. For motion sickness take two capsules of ginger an hour before the trip begins and then every three hours while traveling. I was traveling with some friends to the beach and the one in the back seat was feeling motion sick. I gave her a couple of ginger Altoids from my purse. She was amazed to have her symptoms completely cleared within about 20 minutes and she was able to enjoy the rest of the trip.

For general indigestion drink an herbal tea (1 tsp. of herb per cup of hot water covered and brewed for 10 minutes). The herbs generally most helpful are chamomile, ginger or peppermint (if no GERD).

CASTOR OIL PACKS

Castor oil packs are extremely helpful for a variety of ailments including liver stagnation, stomach and abdominal gas relief, constipation and headaches from stomach distress. Castor oil helps your body heal and discharge toxins. For making a castor oil pack you need the following:

- cotton or wool flannel cloth about 30 inches by three feet
- clear kitchen plastic wrap,
- a glass baking dish (about 9 inches square)
- large bath towel
- two safety pins
- a hot water bottle
- six ounces of castor oil

Pour the castor oil over the flannel folded into the baking dish. Be sure the flannel is well moistened. Lie down and place the oil-soaked flannel on the skin over the abdominal area or area being treated. Place a large piece of plastic wrap over the flannel, so the flannel is covered completely with plastic. Wrap the towel around you, covering everything and pin the towel to itself so it stays in place. Apply a hot water bottle over the flannel. (The hot water bottle should not be applied to the castor oil when there are uterine growths, bleeding, pregnancy, ulcers, while menstruating or if there is a possibility of appendicitis.) Rest -- sleeping or meditating -- for one hour while the pack is on.

After removing the pack, wipe off the oil from the skin and wash with baking soda in water (1 tsp. soda to 1 cup water). You can place the flannel back in the same dish and store in a cool dark place, like the refrigerator, until next time. Add more oil as needed. Each person should use their own pack, not share the same one. This can be done once a day as needed.

DIARRHEA AND VOMITING

Diarrhea and vomiting both occur when the body needs to get rid of a problem – such as during a virus or food poisoning. It is a healthy initial response to eliminating the aggravation. We need to respect that and work with the body as much as possible. For severe cases the first six to twelve hours, no food is best for adults, but plenty of water. This avoids further irritating the linings of the stomach and intestines. When the symptoms have calmed down a bit, try taking clear liquids, such as vegetable broth or diluted juices (half juice and half water) in small sips or teaspoonfuls. Sucking on an ice chip is another way to take in small amounts of fluid. Avoid milk or broth made with oil. Gradually increase the amounts of clear liquids such as juices, broths and jello. Slowly add in foods that are easily digested such as baby food, eggs, canned fruits, cooked vegetables and rice.

An electrolyte replacing drink will frequently be very helpful. These are available at the grocery store in a variety of brands. A quick one to make at home is 6 ounces of water plus 6 ounces of orange juice with a half teaspoon of salt.

Charcoal tablets can be very beneficial if diarrhea continues more than a couple days and is debilitating. It will help absorb and neutralize the toxins. Take two tablets every three hours. Stop after two doses if there is no change in the diarrhea.

Homeopathic Arsenicum album is readily available and very effective for food poisoning where there is both diarrhea and vomiting, the person is restless and thirsty for small sips and/or they have burning pains. Dose as soon as possible, then as needed based on any slight return of symptoms. You should start with a 30C potency and expect some relief of symptoms within about 20 minutes. Repeat as needed. If it does not help at all, stop after three doses; it probably won't help, and you should try a different remedy or treatment. Otherwise continue taking as needed, if it is helping.

CONSTIPATION

Constipation is a general sign that all is not well with your health. The three key items that help you avoid constipation are:

- Regular exercise; walking is good
- Drinking plenty of fluids, especially water

- Eating lots of soluble and insoluble fiber in your diet, such as whole grains, fruits and vegetables, oats and flax meal.

In addition, it is also important to reduce stress through Yoga, Tai Chi, meditation or other stress reducers. If you drink some extra water, go for a walk everyday (which also helps with the stress), have flax meal, chia seeds, whole grains, seeds nuts and lots of fruits and vegetables, you probably won't have a problem.

If occasionally you do have a problem, many people find dried prunes a very helpful addition to the diet. A friend of mine would have problems with constipation whenever he traveled and learned to always take a bag of prunes along on a trip.

Another option that is always available is to gently rub your abdomen clockwise 40 times with the palm of your hand. It also helps diarrhea when you rub counterclockwise to slow down your digestion.

Avoid repeated laxatives and enemas if possible as they are a short-term solution with possible long-term consequences. The herbs Senna and Cascara are very effective ingredients in laxative teas and capsules, but they can become habit forming used long-term. You then have a problem with rebound constipation when you stop them. So only use them acutely for short periods of time.

HEMORRHOIDS

As a result of constipation and straining, people can get hemorrhoids that may be itching, bleeding and painful. Avoiding constipation (see above) and straining are the keys to the long-term cure. Work that requires sitting for long periods should be interrupted every hour or so with some moving around.

If you do have a problem, buy witch hazel-soaked pads at the drug store and apply to the sore area after every bowel movement. Soaking in a sitz bath of warm water helps keep the area clean, improves circulation and soothes the pain. In Chapter 11 I discuss how to do a sitz bath. Using a kinder, gentler toilet paper such as a baby's wet wipes will help clean the area and prevent irritation. A calendula ointment applied to the area can also help speed the healing.

SERIOUS DIGESTIVE CONCERNS

Dehydration is a concern with various illnesses, but especially vomiting and diarrhea. A good way to check for dehydration is to pinch the skin up on the back of the hand and watch to see how fast it falls back to normal. If the skin snaps right back to normal, then the person is probably fine. If a person has tears and saliva then they are probably fine. When someone is dehydrated it is important for them to drink large amounts of fluids, preferably with electrolytes to restore their balance. If they are not able to drink, then it is a medical emergency and they should go to a physician for intravenous therapy.

Constant pain and burning in the stomach area can indicate ulcers. Ulcers are caused by a bacteria, H.Pylori, eating at the lining of the stomach. They are very tolerant of acid and seem to be in many people's stomachs without causing a problem. If your symptoms are mild, chew DGL (De-Glycyrrhizinated Licorice) tablets before each meal and avoid foods that irritate the pain. If you have any black, tarry stools, you need to see a doctor immediately, because you may be bleeding in the upper digestive tract.

Appendicitis pain can be spread out over the abdomen area. If there have been no bowel movements, the abdomen is very tender to touch, and the person is feeling ill, then a doctor needs to be seen as soon as possible for evaluation. Homeopathic Belladonna 30C can be very helpful on the way to being evaluated.

Cancer in the abdominal area can cause a variety of symptoms – change in bowel habits, swelling of the abdomen and palpable new lumps on one side more than the other. Be sure to have any of these symptoms checked out by your doctor.

Celiac Disease is now thought to be a common genetic disease affecting one in one hundred people and of all different nationalities. The common symptoms are from the malabsorption, bleeding and inflammation of the small intestines. In addition, many auto-immune type diseases are caused by Celiac Disease without the obvious diarrhea or constipation issues. If you have been chronically anemic, fatigued, have digestive problems or have allergies you should see your doctor about being assessed for Celiac Disease. There is a longer discussion in Chapter 1 on Celiac Disease.

COLDS AND FLU

An acute illness is a signal from your body telling you to pay attention. Perhaps you need to slow down, rest more and examine your priorities. A cold or flu once a year may also be your body's way of exercising and updating your immune system.

PREVENTION

Homeopathy considers the long-term effect of acute treatment choices. It has become routine to avoid acute illness through whatever means available. But at what cost? At the same time, we have seen a marked increase in suffering from chronic diseases, many of which reflect weaknesses of our immune system. Instead of flu shots, most of us are better off if we let our immune systems go through the more normal course of being exposed to the illness and fighting it off. When the immune system has a healthy workout, it ends up stronger as a result.

You can minimize your susceptibility to cold and flu illnesses if you:

- Include tonic herbs like garlic and ginger in your diet.
- Exercise moderately on a regular basis to keep your circulation at its peak.

- Stay rested and practicing stress reduction techniques such as Tai Chi, Yoga and meditation.
- Wash your hands frequently and avoid touching your eyes and face, especially during flu season.
- Take Echinacea tincture (one dropperful) throughout the cold and flu season as an immune system booster

When you first begin to feel sick, take Vitamin C -- 500 mg two to ten times a day, the mineral ascorbate versions are well absorbed and don't cause diarrhea like the ascorbic acid. Increase your use of Echinacea tincture to three times a day. Eat lightly -- broth soups, vegetable juices and water may be enough.

Hydrotherapy is very effective and available everywhere. You can use it for any of the illnesses described here. The alternating of hot and cold creates a pumping action to move the blood in the body. I had a patient who called me from out of town; he had an important presentation the next day and felt like he was getting ill. I recommended hydrotherapy in the hotel bathtub, alternating hot and cold and then to bed. He reported feeling great the next day. The easy way to do it at home is to fill a dish pan with warm to hot water. Sit down and make yourself comfortable. Soak your feet and ankles for five minutes. Then place your feet in a pan of cold water for a minute and return them to the hot water -- adding more hot water as needed. Repeat this process at least three times. Always finish with the cold. Then dry off your feet, they should be pink and warm. Put on warm, thick socks and lie down and rest for at least twenty minutes.

Antibiotics are often prescribed if a bacterial infection is suspected, but there are at least two problems with antibiotics: 1) They also kill many friendly bacteria in your body. 2) Bacteria have gotten "smarter" and so antibiotics have had to be stronger to be effective.

Antibiotics are not helpful for viral infections. They are wonderful tools for serious bacterial infections when your body is not strong enough to cope. If you take antibiotics, be sure to start a course of probiotics, such as a combination of acidophilus, bifidus and lactobacillus, to repopulate your system as quickly as possible.

SORE THROATS

When your throat is sore, gargling is effective in soothing the irritation. Choose a quarter teaspoon of salt or a quarter teaspoon of Tabasco (cayenne in vinegar) or a dropperful of Echinacea in a cup of warm water. You can alternate these or use whichever one you have on hand. Zinc lozenges can also be very helpful to stop the infection.

Various homeopathic medicines are used frequently for sore throats. If there is a lot of saliva in the mouth with the sore throat, it is probably Mercurius; if the sore throat came on quickly and is very red and sore it could be

Belladonna. Take a 30C dose of the best indicated medicine every 3 hours for three doses, then stop if it has not improved. Continue as needed, if it is helping.

Strep throat is a bacterial throat infection which may be dangerous. If your body heals the infection quickly (in less than a week), then you don't have to worry about the possible risk of rheumatic fever. You should seek medical attention if your sore throat is persistent and severe, and accompanied by a fever, swollen, tender glands under your jaw and you are generally feeling quite ill. Headaches are often experienced with strep throat, but not usually a runny nose or cough.

EARACHES

When you suffer an earache, lay on a hot water bottle using it like a pillow. Fill the hot water bottle with warm, not hot water. Drink lots of water or herbal tea, adding Echinacea and Hypericum tinctures, one dropperful each, three times a day. Gargling with the herbs before swallowing will increase the local relief of the pain.

Another ear pain reliever is mullein oil. Use at body temperature, five drops in the ear. In stores you can find a combination of garlic, mullein and hypericum oils that are very helpful.

Alert: If there has been drainage from the ear, the ear drum could have a hole. If so, do not use the ear drops or anything else directly in the ear.

Homeopathy is very effective in treating ear infections and can help break the repeated cycling that happens in children as their bodies struggle to learn how to heal the infection appropriately. The homeopathic medicine needs to be selected specifically for the symptoms of the person, so a homeopath or naturopath should be consulted. The most common homeopathic remedy I've used for earaches is Pulsatilla – the person is weepy with thick nasal discharge and may be clingy. I give up to three 30C doses every couple hours. If it is helping, then continue. If there is no relief, then stop and see a naturopathic physician.

CONJUNCTIVITIS

Conjunctivitis is an inflammation of the membrane that covers the eyeball and inside of the eyelid. There is redness and a sticky or creamy discharge. It is nicknamed red or pink eye. Follow the recommendations in prevention above for herbs and hydrotherapy.

Itchy eyes can be very distressing, but you can make your own eye wash to sooth them. Use six drops each of Calendula and Hypericum tinctures in ½ cup water that has been boiled and cooled. Store the eye wash in a covered container to keep it clean. Use a clean cotton ball each time you apply the solution. Dip the cotton ball in the solution, then wipe gently across the loosely closed eyelid from the nose to the corner of the eye. Repeat three times, using a clean cotton ball each time. Do this as many times a day as you need to – you can't do it too much.

Homeopathic Euphrasia 30C can be very helpful in many cases. Take a dose every three hours for three doses. Only continue if it is helping. If it is from allergies, homeopathic Pulsatilla will more likely be helpful

If your whole eye becomes quite red seek medical attention immediately. If your eye suddenly becomes red in one small spot, you have probably broken a tiny blood vessel which will heal over after a few days.

COLDS AND FLU

Colds and flu call for bed rest. At the first sign of symptoms do hydrotherapy, increase herbs and Vitamin C and take either homeopathic Aconite 30C or Ferrum Phosphoricum 30C. Aconite tends to be needed when symptoms come on suddenly after a chill. Ferrum Phosphoricum is used for a fever with no other symptoms. If you become ill get plenty of sleep, drink lots of water, herbal teas and juices, eat chicken noodle or garlic soup and stay warm. A fever of up to 103° to 104° F (taken orally) assists your body's defenses and helps it move through the illness quicker and more thoroughly. The runny nose and cough are the body's ways of getting rid of the virus, so don't interfere by taking decongestants. Rather, encourage the natural healing process by drinking lots of fluids, and eating lightly or not at all, blowing your nose, and coughing up phlegm. A vaporizer helps keep everything flowing.

If your nose and the skin around it are tender, use Calendula gel or ointment and switch from tissue to cotton handkerchiefs. There are also tissues with soothing lotion in them. Use an oil or lanolin ointment to protect your skin.

If you tend to be chilly, hot ginger lemonade is a great drink. Grate a two-inch piece of fresh ginger root, add to two cups of water, bring to a boil and simmer covered for ten minutes. Remove it from the heat, strain out the ginger and add the juice of a fresh lemon and one tablespoon of honey. Ginger tea is warming at any time and is particularly helpful when you are ill and deeply chilled. Be sure to store any excess tea in a glass jar in the refrigerator.

At the onset of a cold or flu, drink hot ginger lemonade while you are soaking your feet (as discussed at the beginning of this chapter) to bring on a sweat. After soaking your feet, lie in bed in dry heavy cotton clothes and pile on the covers. This will cause you to sweat profusely. Change your clothes and bedclothes if they are so wet that you feel chilled. Frequently this treatment is enough for complete recovery within a day.

Afterwards be sure to shower away the perspiration on your skin. Inducing a sweat will boost your immune system and speed healing in healthy people, but it is not a good idea for the debilitated, very young, or pregnant women.

SINUSITIS

The first goal of treatment for a sinus congestion is to make your nose run. Getting the mucous out is better than leaving it in. Drink lots of fluids, especially herbal teas that are expectorant (that promote mucous flow). Licorice, Lavender and Chamomile teas are all good expectorant teas. Avoid decongestant teas and medicines which dry up and keep in the discharges.

A face steam can help to clear the sinuses. Boil water and place two tablespoons of loose, dried Lavender or Chamomile in a bowl. Pour the boiling water over the herbs. Sit at a table with the steaming bowl in front of you and put a large towel over your head. Inhale the steam for five to ten minutes. This is both relaxing and clears the sinuses. Repeat as often as needed. After steaming, strain off the herbs and add to your bath water for a soothing soak.

Using hydrotherapy on the face is also very clearing. In the shower alternate hot and cold water on your head and face at least 3 times each. End with the cold water. The pumping action to the blood of the head and face will clear your sinuses.

A Neti pot with saltwater (saline solution) applied regularly can help your sinuses to drain. Quercitin, a supplement, both taken internally and as a homeopathic nasal spray gives many of my patients immediate relief without suppression of the discharge.

Decongestant nose sprays will stop the body's drainage and can prolong the illness and even make it worse if they are used repeatedly. Sinus congestion that persists or becomes severely painful or is accompanied by nausea or dizziness requires medical attention.

Homeopathic Kali bichromium 30C helps many sinus infections, especially when there is a stringy discharge and the pain focus is in one spot. Take 3 doses and if it does not give some relief, stop and consult a homeopath or naturopathic physician. If it does relieve the symptoms, then continue as needed.

COUGHS AND CROUP

A cough is one of the body's ways of ridding itself of mucous. It is generally best to encourage rather than suppress this cleansing process. Try cough drops such as lemon, horehound or anise. Drink plenty of fluids and sip Licorice, Lavender or Chamomile teas. The biggest concern is if the cough is keeping you from sleeping, because sleep is important to healing. Sleep propped up, do an herbal steam before bed, and take an herbal cough syrup to promote a good night's sleep. A simple cough solution can be a teaspoon of honey. Another tip is to press lightly with your finger on your outer throat where the cough is originating and tickling. This can frequently reduce coughing spasms.

Croup is a specific type of barking cough that happens in children under 3 years of age when their small throat swells and spasms. For some children immediate exposure to either cold air outside, or steamy air such as in the bathroom with a hot shower running, will give relief. An herbal steam can also be very helpful – but stay under the towel with the child, both to monitor the temperature and to avoid adding fear. Frequently needed homeopathic medicines for croup are Aconite 30C or Spongia 30C. Aconite is the medicine to choose when the illness comes on quickly, frequently around midnight. A patient who needs Spongia as a medicine has a loud crouping, barking cough. A single dose can quickly relieve their symptoms. Frequently the caregiver can benefit from a dose of Aconite or Rescue Remedy to calm themselves.

If the child can't breathe and there is no cough it is a medical emergency and they need immediate hospital care.

INSOMNIA, STRESS AND HEADACHES

Insomnia, stress and headaches may all be inter-related. Frequently, resolving one can help the others, so you may want to try several of these tips.

INSOMNIA

Insomnia is a huge health problem in our culture. Men on average need 8 hours of sleep a night and women need an average of 8 ½ hours of sleep. Many people do not understand that this is a basic need for good health. Although, there are the rare people who have always slept very little all their lives, have lots of energy and don't need any more. Most people get caught in compensating for their lack of sleep with food or caffeine, which can then keep them from sleeping when they want to, creates a vicious cycle. As the liver slows down, processing caffeine slows, and sleep becomes more of a problem. Not getting enough sleep can cause weight gain. The extra weight sometimes interferes with breathing, adding to the sleep problems.

Sleep researchers have found that many sleep problems resolve by following good sleep habits. Use your bed only for sleeping (and romance, too). Don't watch TV or read exciting books in bed. If you find yourself lying in bed for more than fifteen minutes, waiting to fall asleep get up and do something you don't like doing like reading a boring book. Don't watch the news or work on the computer for at least a half-hour before going to bed. Drink a cup of chamomile or catnip tea for its soothing effects. Some people find taking their calcium and magnesium supplement at bedtime is helpful, but it is important to avoid those B vitamins after dinner because they can keep you awake. If you are just too excited to sleep, then homeopathic Coffea 30C a single dose at bedtime works well.

If insomnia is a consistent problem, plan on having a bedtime routine and regular hours for going to bed and waking. Add vigorous exercise during the day for half an hour, preferably in the morning sun, but before 6 P.M. Being out in the morning sun helps your body produce melatonin. Melatonin is important for going to sleep and some people find success in taking small amounts at bedtime. Avoid caffeinated beverages, especially after noon. If during the afternoon you feel tired – exercise, drink some vitamin C or do some breathing exercises to rejuvenate you.

For more stubborn forms of insomnia I find that there is sometimes a grief component or hormonal imbalance. Having to get up to urinate frequently may be the problem that needs to be addressed. These require evaluation of the individual by a naturopathic physician.

STRESS REDUCTION

Ongoing stress leads to numerous physical problems generally related to adrenal fatigue. The adrenals produce sex and stress hormones for our body. Multiple organ systems in the body can be affected and there can be many different symptoms. The adrenal glands thrive in a life that has a routine for eating and sleeping. They do best with vitamins and minerals acquired from lots of fruits and vegetables in the diet. Having some regular quiet time daily to do yoga, tai chi, qigong, meditation or to pet the cat makes a big difference. The nutrients especially helpful to the adrenals are Vitamin B5 and Vitamin C.

One herb that helps with nervous tension, especially from menopause or premenstrual syndrome is Hypericum (St. John's Wort). You can take the tincture daily in water (one dropperful in 1/4 cup water) or brew a strong tea from the dried flowers. To brew the tea, place one teaspoon in a cup, add boiling water, cover and allow to steep ten minutes. I have a liquid herbal mixture, called Breiten Calming Glycerite, that many of my patients use. It helps calm and gently induce sleep for adults and children. It is made of the liquid glycerite of lavender, passiflora, catnip and oats and works marvelously.

A safe and very effective treatment for anxiety or an emergency is the Bach flower combination called Rescue Remedy. It is a combination of 5 flowering plants that are known for their soothing nature. In a stressful situation, it is amazing how a few drops under the tongue calms kids, pets and adults. I was on a trip with a friend and was caught in a fierce snowstorm coming back down the freeway from Flagstaff, Arizona. She was driving the van and it was one lane of traffic creeping along; visibility was terrible. Suddenly, in a gust of wind, the windshield wiper on the driver's side flew off! Our visibility was almost zero. Miraculously there was a wide spot in the highway, and we were able to get off and stop. She had Rescue Remedy in her purse and we both took a dose. It calmed me down immediately and I could see that all I had to do was get out and move the passenger wiper over to the driver side. Rescue Remedy works very quickly and safely to restore your clarity of thinking. It does not make you sleepy, but I find if someone has been very stressed for a long time they will want to sleep when they calm down. Rescue Remedy can also be placed in a water bottle before a stressful event to drink from, to stay calm and balanced.

Some people have troubles with anxiety as related to stress and many respond well to diet changes. Many times, they are sensitive to carbohydrates and sweets. When they eat them, they feel temporarily better and then an hour or so later can have a panic attack when their blood sugar drops low. Regularly eating a combination of carbohydrate, fat and protein for every meal or snack can reduce these types of anxiety symptoms. An example would be to have peanut butter with an apple or almonds with dried fruit.

HEADACHES

When you have a headache, experiment with other types of pain relief before you pop an aspirin. Immediately drink some extra water, because many headaches are caused by dehydration. Take a short nap; sleep is very restorative. Headaches frequently are the result of sinus infections, migraines, pain in facial nerves or tension and are usually very individual. I find that when someone comes to me with chronic headaches there is not a simple solution because the whole person is involved and has to be treated.

Headache pain may be due to an increase in blood flow in your head. An effective way to reverse the blood flow is to sit with your feet in hot water -- you may notice your hands and feet are cold when you have a headache. Soaking your feet or hands in hot water will move the blood supply away from the head. Placing a cold damp cloth on the back of the neck improve the pain-reducing effects. While you are soaking your feet also apply Lavender essential oil onto your temples.

A good neck massage can help some people. Lie on your back on a firm surface and ask a friend to reach gently under your head and apply steady pressure to the bones at the base of the skull where the neck muscles attach. Rubbing

Arnica ointment or Traumeel ointment on the back of the neck improves the circulation to the nerve nodes which are the source of many headaches.

A very effective herbal combination is to drink a Lavender and Feverfew infusion tea at the first sign of symptoms. To make the tea, use one ounce of Lavender and Feverfew. Place them in a strainer over a cup and add boiling water and cover. Steep for ten minutes then pull out the strainer of herbs. Drink one quarter of a cup at a time as needed. Lavender and feverfew can also be bought in combination as a liquid herbal tincture in many health food stores. Take 20 drops in water at the first sign of pain and then as needed.

Homeopathic treatments for repeat headaches are very individual and the secret of treatment is finding the right medicine for the whole person to become healthier.

Some headaches need immediate attention by your doctor:

- Headaches after an injury to the head.
- Unusual, intense headaches, different from any you have had.
- Headaches accompanied by fever and a neck so stiff you cannot touch your chin to your chest.

ACCIDENTS

Even the healthiest people will have occasional bumps and scrapes. The following are some very effective ways of controlling pain and promoting healing.

BRUISES AND SPRAINS

The most frequent types of injuries are bruises, muscle strains and sprains.

Arnica ointment is remarkable. It eases bruise pain immediately and can reduce the discoloration if used right away. For bruises from bumping into something, rub Arnica ointment onto the sore spot. If you have achy muscles from overdoing a physical activity, try ice packs in combination with the Arnica ointment. Don't use Arnica ointment if there is broken skin, as it will irritate the open wound. A bag of frozen peas or corn work as an emergency ice pack and will wrap around the sore spot easily.

Homeopathic medicines are usually found in stores where natural products are sold. You will find several different potencies of homeopathic Arnica available. The lower potencies, such as 6C, 12C and 30C are for smaller events, minor accidents and falls. The higher strength 200C now available in many stores is for more extensive damage. For example, one evening my mother and I were walking through the high school parking lot to my daughter's choir performance. Mom didn't see the speed bump in the dark, tripped on it and fell to the ground. She was embarrassed and jumped right up, so nothing appeared to be broken. I gave her 200C Arnica from my purse, 3 pellets, gave her the tube to put in her pocket with instructions to take another dose if it started hurting again. The next day she gave the tube back to me and reported that she had only needed one additional dose during the show and had no soreness or bruising from the fall. This is a good example where an immediate dose of Arnica kept her body from going into the bruising, congestion and soreness we would normally associate with a fall to the ground.

I recommend starting with Arnica ointment. You can't overuse it and it works great on bruises and sore muscles. Then evaluate if homeopathic pellets are necessary. The pellets are more powerful and the higher the number on the tube the more powerful. It is best to dose matching the severity with the potency. If you are sore from a strenuous work out, 30C probably will do the trick. If you had a bad fall or car accident, you will need 200C or maybe higher to control pain and swelling.

When there is bleeding and bruising together, use the plant Yarrow (Achillea millefolium) fresh or in a tincture or a salve on the injury. Dilute the Yarrow tincture one dropperful to one-quarter cup of water and pour it on a bandage so the pad is soaked with the tincture. Place it over the wound. If you have fresh Yarrow, crush the fresh leaves and stems, then apply directly to the wound. It will speed healing, reduce pain, and stop bleeding.

For a sprained ankle or other sprain, remember **R**est, **I**ce, **C**ompression and **E**levation or **RICE** and apply Arnica ointment. Stop to rest, apply an ice pack, gently wrap the sprain in an Ace bandage and elevate the sprain. Reapply the Arnica if the pain returns and continue to rest. You will need extra rest to help your body heal. For very serious sprains, homeopathic Arnica 30C is very effective for both pain relief and speeding the healing. With a sprained ankle, excessive swelling may indicate how many of the supporting structures have been damaged in the sprain. Avoid standing on it until the pain is decreased. A splint may be needed to support your ankle until the ligaments heal.

When a nerve rich area like the fingers, toes, lips, nose, ears or coccyx is bruised it is usually accompanied by shooting pains. Use Hypericum in homeopathic, oil or tincture. Apply the oil at once directly on the skin and the pain will usually stop on contact. (Hypericum is commonly known as St. John's Wort.) Next apply some Hypericum oil or tincture to a bandage or gauze and put it over the damaged area. If the skin is cut or broken, dilute the tincture first in water (twenty drops in one-quarter cup of water). The undiluted alcohol in the tincture will sting and irritate if there is broken skin. Pour the mixture over the injury or soak the finger or toe in it. Hypericum stops the pain, is antimicrobial and promotes rapid healing. For ongoing nerve pain, add a dose of homeopathic Hypericum 30C under the tongue.

When there is broken skin over any severe injury, but particularly over fingers where the bones are close to the surface, it is important to know if the bone underneath is broken. If the cause of injury was very forceful and the finger won't move without a lot of pain, an x-ray may be necessary. If you can find one small spot that is very tender, especially with bruising and swelling, there may be a fracture. Seek medical attention to help decide if an x-ray is needed.

CUTS

Wash cuts and burns gently and thoroughly with soap and water before treatment. Cover them as needed to protect the wound and keep it clean. If there is excessive bleeding, apply a drop of calendula tincture to the wound and a clean dry dressing and hold with slight pressure. You will be amazed at how quickly the bleeding will stop and how fast the cut will heal.

One day Ric cut his index finger very deeply while washing dishes — a glass broke as he inserted his hand into the water. A dropperful each Calendula and Hypericum herbal tinctures mixed into a 1/4 cup of water were poured over the cut. This sped the healing and relieved the bleeding and nerve pain. A clean pad applied to the cut with gentle pressure also helped control the bleeding. A splint was necessary for a few days to keep the finger from moving and reopening the wound.

Later, he soaked his fingers in water and Calendula and Hypericum tinctures when the cut began to hurt again. The pain stopped immediately. His finger healed beautifully and completely.

For puncture wounds, begin by gently pressing around the wound to encourage bleeding. Homeopathic Ledum 30C, works well with puncture wounds to speed complete healing. Wash the cut with soap and water as soon as possible, apply some Calendula and take a dose of Ledum under your tongue.

A small border of redness (1/4") around a healing wound is a healthy sign of the body's work.

Warning: A large area of redness, red streaking going up the arm or leg, marked tenderness in the area, or yellow or green drainage, each can indicate a possible infection and needs medical attention as soon as possible.

BURNS AND SUNBURN

Hypericum oil is nice for preventing sunburn if the sun is not too intense. Of course, there are lots of sunscreens on the market to choose from. I prefer those that are considered safe for children and are all natural. Apply something to your skin before you go out between 10:00 AM and 2:00 PM when the sun's rays are most dangerous. Protecting your skin can keep you looking younger and reduce the chances of skin cancer. [Getting sun in the early morning or evening can be a great source of Vitamin D, so don't use sunscreen 100% of the time.] I have had good success with Hypericum oil topically on my sunburn; it stopped the pain and sped the healing.

Where blistering doesn't occur it is usually a first degree burn and you can treat with Hypericum or Calendula tincture diluted (one dropperful to 1/4 cup cool water) and sprayed from a clean spray bottle or splashed onto the burn. Aloe vera is a great plant to keep in the kitchen for burns of any kind. Split open a leaf of the aloe vera plant and apply the slimy gel-like substance all over the burnt area. You can also purchase aloe vera gels, read the ingredient label carefully to be sure it is mostly aloe vera. Green tea has worked well on sunburns at our house if the burns are not too severe. We brew it up and when the tea cools splash or spray it on.

Homeopathic Urtica urens 30C or Cantharis 30C under the tongue can be very helpful in speeding healing and reducing pain. Urtica is for the hot, but not so painful burn. Cantharis is for the very painful burn, sometimes blistering. One day I was in my car and I pulled my cell phone charger out of the cigarette lighter and replaced the cigarette lighter. As I was driving along, it suddenly popped out which surprised me and I leaned over to pick it up. Unfortunately, it had heated up and I burned my index finger pad in a neat circle. Boy did it hurt! I sucked on it as I drove along and that helped a little. I put an ice cube on it when I got home and it helped, but as soon as I took it off it started hurting again. It blistered in a nice circle. I took a dose of homeopathic Cantharis 200C and the pain stopped completely. I took another dose at bedtime and in the morning, I awoke to a circle on my finger, but no blister and no pain. It never bothered me again.

Ice applied promptly to a burn is always a good idea to reduce the pain. Don't break blisters if you can avoid it, because when intact they protect from infection. Avoid greasy ointments and creams that retain the heat. When you are burned drink plenty of fluids, with the exception of alcohol or caffeinated beverages, as they are dehydrating. Get extra rest to give your body support and promote healing.

1   First degree burn: red, sensation to a pinprick

2   Second degree burn: red to pink to white, often with blisters, pinprick sensation

3   Third degree burn: leathery, white, black or brown, no pinprick sensation

If there are signs of second degree burn over 25% of the body or third degree burn over 10% it is a medical emergency and the patient must be taken to a burn center.

CALMING AND SHOCK PREVENTION

When accidents occur, calming the people involved is vital to restoring order. In this situation, I recommend a Bach flower combination, Rescue Remedy. It contains a mixture of five flowers that are helpful in emotional emergencies. Reach for a few drops when people or pets are feeling shaky after an accident, even if there is no apparent damage. If Rescue Remedy isn't quite enough, then homeopathic Aconite 30C can relieve the fear and calm the person.

One day I had a young woman come into my office at the college where I was working, whose car had gone off the road down into a creek bed. She was chilled, wrapped in a blanket, but not hurt, was mildly confused and looking for a friend. I asked her if I could give her a dose of Aconite and she said yes. After the dose, she immediately got focused, needed to sit down and was shortly able to move on with her business. Interestingly, when I patted her on the back as she left, it now radiated heat.

For the people injured in an accident, the homeopathic remedy Arnica 30C or 200C will reduce the risk of going into shock.

STINGS AND BITES

In a healthy person insect bites or bee stings present few problems beyond some mild discomfort. However, if there is a severe response, such as difficulty breathing, it could be an allergic reaction and life threatening. The crucial factor is whether a reaction occurs at a place separate from the sting. If you are having swelling in other areas of the body, especially a sensation of swelling in your throat, with a sense of unease, this is an emergency and you should go to the Emergency Room. If you are stung on your finger, your whole arm may swell, and be uncomfortable, but this is unlikely to be dangerous. If you are stung on your finger and your other hand starts to swell, it is affecting your circulatory system. You should seek immediate medical attention. Homeopathic Apis 30C is effective in reducing the reaction while you are in transit.

Carefully remove any visible stinger with tweezers grabbing close to the skin. (Using your fingers can squeeze more of the irritant under the skin.) Relieve the itching and inflammation of stings by applying ice, cold compresses and a baking soda paste. Calendula tincture (one dropperful to one-quarter of a cup water) or Calendula cream, placed on the bite or sting will reduce the discomfort. Arnica ointment is also helpful.

There is a natural product called SssstingStop. It comes in a tube, is easy to carry, and is applied topically to the sting or bite. It works quickly and effectively. When nothing else is available, use the onion remedy. Place the cut side of half an onion on the sting to relieve the pain.

A bite from a poisonous spider should be packed in ice to slow down the spread of the poison. The homeopathic remedy Ledum 30C can frequently be very helpful. Go to the nearest hospital. If possible, bring the spider so it can be identified.

With an insect sting the greatest risk is a severe allergic reaction.

One day in Puerto Penasco, Mexico, my 13-year-old daughter Jo, was stung by a stingray on the top of her foot in the ocean surf. It was intense pain and a big surprise. My other daughter, Lili, and I formed a chair with our hands and carried her back to shore. I gave her a dose of homeopathic Lachesis from my first aid kit. This helped her feel well enough to be able to walk the considerable distance back to our rental house. Stingray venom is a unique venom which detoxifies in hot water. At the house we soaked her foot in water as hot as she could stand. It stopped most of the pain and the wound went from purple to red. With a dose of homeopathic Apis she was feeling like playing again and it was just a little over an hour since the sting!

She was fine until about a week later when her foot became inflamed, swollen and painful again, probably from bacteria deep in the puncture wound. A treatment combination of homeopathic Hepar sulphuris calcareum 30C under her tongue, drinking herbal Echinacea tincture in water plus hydrotherapy (soaking her foot in hot water with Epsom salt alternating with cold water) several times a day cleared up the infection permanently in two days.

Stings and bites have long been treated with herbal Echinacea by Native Americans. Echinacea should be applied topically on the wound and taken internally as a tea made from the root. I've applied Echinacea tincture topically to a jelly fish sting and it stopped hurting immediately.

SUNSTROKE

You can prevent heat illness from over exposure to the sun by wearing a hat and drinking plenty of water and consuming adequate salt to replace what you are losing in your perspiration. Avoid caffeinated and alcoholic beverages when you are out in the sun because they can add to dehydration. Keep an eye out for the early signs of headache, dizziness and weakness.

If you begin to feel the signs of sunstroke, such as headache, dizziness, nausea, diarrhea and you are no longer sweating, lie down in as cool a place as you can find and make your own electrolyte drink by diluting fruit juice half with water, one cup each and adding a half teaspoon of salt. Soak a cloth in room-temperature water and place it on your head while resting. Homeopathic Glonoinum 30C under the tongue speeds recovery.

HEAD INJURIES

Traumas to the head, like a blunt hit from fainting, a car accident or a hard fall to the ground, can cause concussions. One of the serious concerns is that the brain might swell from a bruising response. If someone has been unconscious, their eyes are not equally dilated or they are not able to accurately answer questions, they need to be checked out by a physician. Homeopathic Arnica 200C can keep the brain from swelling after an injury. Frequently homeopathic Natrum sulphuricum 30C will be required during recovery, especially if the patient was unconscious for very long or they are unusually depressed after the head injury.

A neighbor of mine hit his head on the ice while playing hockey. He hit it very hard twice in a row as his head bounced. He was hospitalized for several days, then released, but was still unable to take care of himself or remember basic information. His wife came to me after a few days asking for help. A single dose of homeopathic Hypericum 200C helped him recover totally within a couple of hours.

Injuries to the eyes respond well to homeopathic Aconite 30C. It is like the Arnica of the eyes, take it after any blow to the eye for rapid assistance in reducing pain and healing.

For minor eye injuries, mix 1 teaspoon Calendula tincture in a ¼ cup of sterile water, dip a cotton ball in the mixture and wipe the closed eye, one time per each cotton ball, from the inside corner to the outside. This will help speed healing and prevent infection.

Homeopathic Phosphorus 30C works quickly and well to stop nose bleeds. Nosebleeds from a hit to the nose can generate a lot of bright red blood. Applying external pressure to the root of the nose can be helpful. Keep the head forward so the blood is not swallowed. Repeat the Phosphorus as needed, keep the person quiet until the bleeding has been securely stopped for awhile.

FRACTURES

Broken bones have to be evaluated by a physician and then immobilized for healing. Some Arnica for the initial pain is helpful – give the highest potency you have and repeat as needed to control the initial pain. To speed the healing and control the discomfort there are two additional homeopathic remedies I use. Calcarea phosphoricum 30C in the morning and Symphytum 30C in the evening. They are best not taken together, but should be taken for several months to speed the healing of the broken bone. Make sure to eat a diet with lots of fruits, vegetables and protein while recovering.

SKIN CARE

The skin is frequently a reflection of what is taking place inside the digestive tract. The intestinal lining and the skin are all epithelial cells. So, what is happening to one is probably also happening elsewhere. Therefore, very healthy skin usually indicates great digestion. The skin also is a major inlet and outlet of the body for detoxification.

What we put on our scalp, our skin or place our hands into should be the same quality as what we eat. Look carefully at labels of shampoos, cream rinses, lotions and deodorants to assess the ingredients. Avoid aluminum, and artificial colors. I chose organic, herbal products and am very pleased with the wonderful variety there is to chose from and how well they work.

When we perspire or have a skin eruption, we are activating a route of elimination of toxins from the body. In treating skin problems, it is important not to suppress the body's process of elimination. Suppression is recognized when a skin problem goes away, but a more serious internal problem develops or gets worse. A good rule of thumb is not to directly dry up any discharges or secretions with medications. These are the body's way of removing problems.

Instead, try to speed up, or bring the discharge to a head so it can heal naturally. Most importantly, treat the root of the problem.

If your skin tends to be dry, you can soften and lubricate the skin topically by applying non-scented, hypoallergenic lotions, Calendula ointment or Almond oil, Coconut oil, Olive oil or Lanolin oil as needed. Right after washing or a shower is an especially good time to apply oils to help retain the moisture in your skin. Occasionally dry skin along with being chillier, losing hair and more fatigue can indicate hypothyroid issues and should be checked by your physician.

Oily skins benefit from cleansing with water and then an astringent application like apple-cider vinegar, witch hazel or lemon water. Soaps, if the skin is not actually dirty, can be too harsh on the face; just use water and your washcloth.

Witch hazel can also be helpful if you wake up with puffy eyes. Soak a cotton ball in the witch hazel and pat it around your eyes where they are puffy.

Help your skin be healthier. Eat nuts, seeds, olive oil, or coconut oil for good fatty acids. Drink plenty of water so you are hydrated to help your skin look smoother. Smoking can also create a lot of wrinkles and speeds aging of the skin.

When your lips are dry and chapped, Calendula gel or ointment works wonderfully well and you will be surprised how little you need. Be aware of chap stick, as some brands make your lips feel better immediately, but over the long run dry your lips. I have found the organic and herbal ones don't have that effect. Look for Calendula or Aloe in the ingredient list of a lip balm, to help your lips heal.

POISON OAK

Poison oak is an allergy reaction of your skin to the oils from the poison oak or ivy plant. After exposure, immediately wash the skin to remove the oils with half dish soap and half water then rinse well. Don't use a washcloth because the oil can get on it and spread the poison oak oils to other parts of the body. Carefully remove and wash clothes in hot water. Tecnu is a product you can buy which also effectively removes the oils causing the irritation. If you have a new eruption after initial treatment, clean again, because you did not get all of the oils the first time.

After a rash has developed, the main complaint is generally itching. Cold compresses or a little rubbing alcohol on the itchy spot can help. Another helpful tip is to wet a Tylenol or aspirin tablet then rub it on the itchy area or you can take a baking soda and apple cider vinegar bath for relief. Green clay is another product you can purchase to help draw out and dry the rash.

Homeopathic Rhus toxicondron 30C can be very helpful in relieving symptoms, especially if the itching is better after a very hot shower. Take every couple of hours as needed.

COLD SORES

Cold sores are a frequent skin problem for many people. They generally appear during times of stress, fatigue or infection. Cold sores begin as a painful or tingling sensation and need to be treated as soon as you are aware of the feeling. lavender oil, 10 drops -- in one ounce of plain oil such as olive oil -- and applied as soon as possible and repeated frequently, will prevent the cold sore. Cayenne, as in a Tabasco type sauce from the kitchen, will work if dabbed on the spot as soon as possible. Melissa officinalis and chaparral (Larrea tridentata) are herbs known to be very effective topically and can be purchased in natural stores. The amino acid, L-Lysine, taken in pill form, helps to prevent cold sores.

Canker sores inside the mouth are a problem for many people and will be helped by goldenseal (Hydrastis canadensis) tincture (50 drops in ½ cup water). Rinse your mouth and spit it out three to four times a day for three or four days. Some commercial mouthwashes, like Listerine, have Thyme extract in them as an active ingredient. They are very helpful in reducing inflammation and infection.

ACNE

Pimples and acne heal faster if you keep the skin clean, eat well and leave it alone. If the pimple is very sore, hot cloths just to the sore spot can help it come to a head so it will drain and dry up. Another approach is to rub a clove of fresh garlic onto the affected area at bedtime. You could do it during the day too, if others don't object. I have found that chaparral with calendula applied to a pimple speeds the healing.

For cystic acne, a very painful type of acne, homeopathic Hepar sulphuris calcareum 30C taken daily, is very helpful in reducing pain and swelling.

The primary issue for acne is the health of the digestive tract. Open all the other routes of elimination and heal the gut to improve the skin without suppression. This can mean testing for allergens in the diet, diet changes, liver cleanse and making sure there is plenty of water intake, fiber intake and exercise. Hormonal imbalances can also contribute. A naturopathic physician can be very helpful in determining the cause of the problem.

ATHLETE'S FOOT

Sometimes athlete's foot is just unattractive, other times it is unattractive and uncomfortable. Apply undiluted apple cider vinegar directly after each shower or Vick's Vapor Rub applied after the vinegar has been shown to reduce fungus. Always dry your foot thoroughly before putting on shoes and socks. This treatment can be repeated as often as necessary and the vinegar will help to dry out the athlete's foot and make you more comfortable. Go barefoot as much as possible to give the foot air and keep it dry.

Sometimes athlete's foot is the body's way of discharging – we heal from the top down, the inside out and most serious to least serious. The discharges on the feet can be the last to heal.

MEASLES, MUMPS AND CHICKEN POX

These are all diseases that exercise the immune system. In children they are a time to be quiet and stay home, but generally are not serious. In general, the appetite is decreased with all three. Respect the appetite and eat basic, nutritious foods in small quantities. Encourage fluids, especially if there is a fever, to avoid dehydration.

Especially with chicken pox it is important to try to keep the patient from scratching the sores, to avoid scarring. Trim the fingernails as short as possible to minimize damage from involuntary scratching. Try to avoid breaking the blisters or disturbing the scabs. Never give aspirin to a child with chicken pox because it is believed to help trigger Reyes Syndrome, a life-threatening illness. A baking soda or oatmeal bath will soothe the itching (add one cup of baking soda to the bath tub of water or for oatmeal, place it in a fine mesh bag like a big tea bag).

Homeopathic remedies will help mitigate the symptoms; the trick is you have to find the right one, so check with a professional.

DERMATITIS

Food allergies are frequently involved as the root of the problem in dermatitis. Identifying and eliminating them is fundamental to allowing the body to heal. Eating foods we are allergic to can be like a cut you keep poking at. When the gut is inflamed, the skin is inflamed. The intestines and the skin are all epithelial cells, so what we see on the skin is also frequently going on inside the digestive tract. Homeopathic treatment is frequently helpful in assisting the body to heal when allergens are removed. Herbal medicines can be helpful in some cases, but if there are many allergies and a person is very environmentally sensitive, then there frequently are sensitivities to herbs also.

An itchy, red rash commonly known as eczema can be inflamed and uncomfortable. Calendula tincture (one dropperful in ¼ cup water) is very healing to the skin. Splash it on several times a day. Wear only cotton clothing next to the skin. Be sure to thoroughly rinse all of your clothes when you wash them to get rid of any soap residue. Use the minimum soap possible on the skin and avoid very hot baths and showers as they can trigger the itch. If the skin is dry, a bland, unmedicated lotion or cream such as Olive oil, Coconut oil or Lubriderm can be used. Avoid corticosteroid -- hormone creams --

if possible. Corticosteroids when they clear the skin can cause the reaction to go into deeper levels like asthma. It is not unusual for people with skin allergies to develop asthma after corticosteroid treatment.

For weeping and oozing problems, cold compresses can be soothing and a cold milk compress, is especially good. Calamine lotion can be used to dry it out but avoid brands with menthol added as an ingredient.

FROSTBITE

Frostbite is a serious ailment from overexposure to cold of your fingers, nose or toes from being in freezing cold weather or large freezers too long. The fingers or toes will have no feeling and can be white colored. Do not thaw until you are out of the cold as thawing and refreezing can cause more damage.

The initial method of thawing and warming the toes or fingers makes a large difference in the outcome. Warm the frozen part very gently in warm (not hot) water or hold the frozen part against warm skin to re-warm. Holding it in your hands can work well. The re-warming can be very painful as the circulation re-establishes itself in the frozen area. Too rapid warming, like exposing the affected part next to a hot fire or very hot water, can damage the tissues, so take it very slowly.

ABSCESSES

Abscesses can occur anywhere on the body where an infection has closed itself off instead of draining. They can be very painful. The teeth are especially difficult to drain. Alternating hot and cold-water soaks is very effective in bringing more blood into the area and helping the body discharge – but it is tough to soak your head if it is a tooth or on your face. Hot cloths applied topically, with a hot water bottle behind it, are usually very helpful in reducing pain. I don't recommend a heating pad because the dry, electrical heat does not have the same effect as the moist heat.

I use one of two homeopathic medicines when dealing with abscesses. Silicea 30C for an abscess that is clearly a problem but is not exquisitely painful or Hepar sulphuris calcareum 30C when the abscess responds very well to heat and is extremely painful. I repeat the remedies only three times every few hours, if it is not helpful stop or move to the other one. If it is helping, then repeat as needed to control the pain and encourage a discharge.

Echinacea frequently is very helpful as a blood cleanser to support the body's healing of an abscess. If it is a tooth, add to your treatment herbal hypericum tincture and calendula tincture. Twenty drops of each in a ¼ cup of water is plenty. Swish and swallow several times per day to relieve pain and encourage lymphatic drainage of the area.

Fresh aloe vera officinalis plant, found in many plant stores, is a great healer to have in the house. Apply it to a burn, cut, sore or inflamed gums in your mouth. To prepare, cut off a 2 to 3-inch piece from one stem of the plant. Peel it so that all of the green skin is off and only the clear inner gel remains. It is important to remove all the green – it can be upsetting to your stomach. Apply it to the area needing to heal. For dental problems, tuck a chunk of clear aloe gel into your cheek next to your sore spot and leave it there for several hours.

URINARY TRACT AND PROSTATE

HEALTHY URINARY TRACT

Avoid urinary tract infections (UTI) by always drinking plenty of water. Caffeinated, alcoholic and sugar drinks can both irritate the bladder and dehydrate you. Be sure to go to the bathroom as soon as you have the urge and after sexual contact, bike rides and horseback riding type of activities.

Women and girl's extra precautions:

- Avoid bubble baths, vaginal sprays and colored or scented toilet paper.
- Wipe from front to back after going to the bathroom, so the bacteria in the colon are not carried into the urinary tract area.
- Wear 100% cotton underpants. Avoid tight pants.

URINARY TRACT INFECTION

An infection in the urinary tract needs prompt attention. It generally starts in the bladder and is not too serious there, but if the bacteria travel up the ureter tubes to the kidneys, then we have a very serious illness. If the infection is affecting the kidneys, a tap to the back over the lower rib cage will be so painful the patient will jump. In addition to the back pain, chills and high fever are all signs of needing immediate medical care because the infection has spread to the kidneys.

Some of the early signs of a UTI include more frequent urination, painful urination or abdominal pain, urgency to urinate or an inability to hold the urine. Women and girls are most frequently affected. One of the first things you want to do when there are early signs of an acute urinary tract infection is to increase water intake to where the urine color is quite pale. Keeping the water flowing down the tubes from the kidneys to the bladder helps prevent the infection from spreading up to the kidneys. Drinking unsweetened Cranberry juice in water is an excellent choice as the cranberry juice also helps the body's defenses. Cranberries interfere with the most common UTI bacteria's ability to attach to the bladder, making the bacteria easier to wash out and keep from multiplying. Add Vitamin C to boost your immune system and acidify your urine.

Doing sitz baths once or twice a day is also very helpful to the body in clearing the infection. Find two tubs of water you can sit in with your legs hanging out. Fill one with hot, the other with cold water. Sit first in the hot 5 minutes, then the cold water a couple minutes, alternating three times, ending with the cold. If this clears the symptoms, then continue the cranberry and

Vitamin C for an additional day and you are probably fine.

When you don't catch it early enough or it is not responding quickly to the cranberry and Vitamin C, then additional herbs and homeopathic treatments need to be added. Urinary herbal combinations available at the store which include Uva ursi, Oregon grape root and marshmallow root can be very effective. The first day of the infection take a double dose. The second day and at least a day after symptoms clear, take the recommended dose. I prefer tinctures in water which are rapidly absorbed, but capsules with lots of water work well for many people. Uva ursi does not work well with cranberry juice so use one or the other.

Some common homeopathic remedies include Sarsaparilla, Pulsatilla and Cantharis. I would recommend that you consult with your naturopathic physician to differentiate the symptoms if you do not have a homeopathic Materia Medica to refer to.

BLADDER CONTROL

Bladder control is something that many women have difficulty with after childbirth. Pelvic muscle exercises, called Kegel exercises, strengthen the group of muscles in the pelvic floor. When these muscles are weak, urine can leak. Regular exercise of these muscles can improve bladder control. To know which muscle to exercise, try to stop or slow the stream of urine as you are urinating. You are also exercising the right muscle if it also squeezes the vaginal muscle and the anus as when you try not to pass gas. If you are able to stop the urine you will know it is the right muscle. Remember, don't tense the abdominal, buttock or thigh muscles. Be sure to breathe while doing the exercise – don't hold your breath.

Five times a day do a set by squeezing this muscle for a slow count of three and then relax completely for a slow count of three, repeating ten times for one set. Some women do them at every stop light while driving, some when they get up, at breakfast, lunch and dinner, then at bedtime.

BEDWETTING FOR CHILDREN

Bedwetting for children is considered normal until the child is six or so. Even after that age, it may clear up without treatment. Nighttime bladder control is something that takes considerable brain development, so the child may not be neurologically ready yet. when bedwetting stops, then reoccurs in children, it may be a stress response.

When bedwetting recurs or goes beyond six years of age, it may be caused by a wide range of stresses including infection, food allergies or sensitivities, a new home, parental separation or a new sibling. Products like pull-on, panty-style diapers can reduce the clean-up frustrations in the middle of the night for the parent and child. It is very unlikely that the child is doing this deliberately. Compassion and assistance work much better than anger or shaming.

If there is no apparent cause, then evaluate the child's diet and remove the possible foods known to cause these problems. Milk, citrus fruits and chocolate are frequently implicated. Allergy testing, especially for Immunoglobulin G (IgG) antibodies can speed the identification of personal culprit foods.

Avoid powerful drugs if possible since this could suppress symptoms without resolving the underlying problem. Rather, see a naturopathic physician or a homeopath for evaluation of the child. The correct constitutional homeopathic medicine will assist the child in the development and healing necessary for bladder control while sleeping.

MEN'S PROSTATE HEALTH

Many men over forty begin to have problems with their prostate gland. A common condition known as Benign Prostatic Hypertrophy (BPH) can cause an enlargement of the prostate which may interfere with urination. Other symptoms include an increased urgency to urinate with a need to get up in the middle of the night to urinate. Sometimes there is a split stream of urine or an incomplete emptying of the bladder. Eating an organic and high-fiber diet with good fats is very important. Studies have shown that men who eat five to ten servings a day of fruits and vegetables regularly throughout their lives are not as likely to have BPH. It appears that pesticides and contaminants may concentrate in the sex organs, so eating lots of organic fruits and vegetables abundant in protective, health enhancing nutrients will improve the quality of your life in several ways.

An herbal prostate formula can be very helpful for improving the health and function of the prostate. It can encourage pelvic drainage, thereby enhancing the clearance of toxins from the prostate. Look for formulas which include Saw Palmetto, Nettles root, Raspberry leaf and in addition to other herbs. A healing response would be less interrupted sleep, less urgency and better energy within a week or two on the formula.

When the prostate becomes inflamed and infected, it is called prostatitis. This can be painful and will probably require a physician's assessment and possibly antibiotics. During an infection, alternating hot and cold packs or doing hot and cold sitz baths two or three times a day will help circulation to the area and promote healing.

There is concern about cancer of the prostate for many men. It is felt that slow growing forms of prostate cancer are present in most men that live to an old age. There is a current debate whether there is any advantage to treating this with radiation or chemotherapy, since it can possibly negatively affect quality of life and increase the aggressiveness of the cancer. Discuss your options with a naturopathic physician in addition to your urologist.

MENSTRUAL CONCERNS

Women have a different cycle to their life than men as menstrual time clearly demonstrates. It is intended to be a time when life is a little slower and quieter. After menses women are then often full of energy and able to accomplish a lot. Just before, during and after the menses, pre-menstrual, women's intuition can be especially strong and closer to the surface.

Many women suffer from cramping pain with their menses. The homeopathic remedy, Magnesium phosphoricum 30C every few hours is generally very helpful in relieving this pain. In addition, for acute pain, twenty drops in water of the herb crampbark (Viburnum opulus) tincture, every fifteen minutes for several hours, then reduced to four times a day is very helpful in stopping menstrual cramping pain. A hot water bottle over the uterus and some rest can also work wonders. The menses are an important monthly discharge helping to keep women healthy through their child-bearing years. It is not normal for the menses to be an extended length, extremely heavy flow or very painful.

Emotional can sometimes be very strong in women just prior to menses. These symptoms are helped by taking a multi-vitamin and mineral supplement that includes a complement of the B vitamins plus minerals like magnesium and selenium. Taking some quiet time to do yoga, qigong or to meditate can also be very helpful. This is a time of the month when the emotional issues are closer to the surface and need to be acknowledged and processed.

Peri-menopause and menopause is the time when the natural process of a woman's menstrual flow stops. Women are returning to the hormone balance they had when they were young girls before puberty when estrogen was not as dominant a hormone. The adrenal glands produce sex hormones, cortisol and adrenalin. These last two hormones play a huge part in how we react to stress. If a woman has had a very stressful life, the adrenal glands don't do a very good job of becoming the major producer of sex hormones at menopause. Stressed out women are more prone to menopausal symptoms such as hot flashes and mood swings for this reason.

Adrenal health is improved with regular sleep, eating balanced meals routinely and exercising consistently.

PET HEALTH

PETS

To improve the health of a pet, understanding their breed's natural way of eating and imitating it can greatly improve their health. For example, dogs are animals whose stomachs are made to eat regularly, so although they will get overweight if you overfeed them, it does not affect them in other ways like it does cats. Cats in the wild eat every couple of days when they kill an animal – so their stomach acid is designed to work periodically. If cats are eating all the time, then the constant stomach acid can be damaging to their digestive system and kidneys, resulting in sensitive skin and a poor coat. Many people have cats on constant dry food. Feeding them only once or twice a day will greatly improve their mood, their coat, reduce dander and keep them at a healthy weight.

Certainly, feeding animals fresh food with some vitality in it will also improve their health. Some people prepare raw foods for their animals to eat every day and I applaud them. It takes extra time but is highly beneficial for the animals.

Animals are here to work beside us in our lives – they make us laugh, they adjust the energies around us, and they reflect our issues to us.

TREATMENT OPTIONS

Animals experience the same positive response to homeopathic remedies that people do. Cows, sheep, horses, birds, dogs and cats are all being treated successfully with homeopathy. It is simply trickier to determine an animal's state and find the right remedy. A good animal communicator can frequently help in understanding what they are feeling experiencing. There are homeopathic veterinarians available around the country and they use the same homeopathic books and symptoms that we use with people. The questions they will ask will be similar to those you are asked by your homeopath. Study your animal closely before calling so you will be prepared.

Chronic antibiotics, cortisone, vaccinations and stress can make your animal ill. Itchy skin problems in a dog and vomiting in a cat may be evidence of an unhealthy response to vaccinations. These are signs their vital force is weak. The appropriate homeopathic remedies along with a natural and appropriate diet of raw foods can restore your pet to radiant health. After vaccination many dogs need the homeopathic remedy Thuja 30C and cats generally do better with the homeopathic remedy Silicea 30C.

Acupuncture and chiropractic work very well on animals when indicated. Veterinarians now are training in these specialties to provide effective symptom and pain relief.

Herbal medicine does not work the same with animals. Different animal types have unique nutritional needs and ability to process certain substances. However, most animals do well when applying the same concepts of fresh foods, plenty of fiber and good fats to their diet. I have had numerous patients tell me I am prescribing the same supplement their vet has recommended for their animal. A good example is flax- seed; it seems to be good for owners and pets both.

TRAVEL WITH PETS

Traveling with a pet can be an interesting experience. Some animals do not travel well and so their owners give them strong sedatives for the trip. This does have some risks for their health but is better than having them upset the whole way.

An alternative natural treatment without the side effects is a few pellets of Aconite 30C or a couple drops of Rescue Remedy in any water they drink while traveling. It is very effective in reducing the fear level, which seems to be the main cause of problems. They are then able to travel calmly, and everyone can enjoy the trip.

Be sure they are comfortable with the crate you are taking them in. Go on a trial run in the car to get them used to the idea and for you to see that all will work as intended.

If you are not going to take them with you, be sure to tell them you are leaving and that you will return to them, so they know you are not abandoning them or giving them away.

TRAVEL TIPS

Before you go traveling, assemble a small kit of essentials for emergencies. Include the following in your first aid kit: Ginger capsules, Echinacea capsules or tincture, Calendula tincture, Hypericum oil, Arnica ointment and Rescue Remedy. In addition, take the following homeopathic remedies in 30C potency: Aconitum napellus, Arnica Montana, Arsenicum album and Cocculus.

Ginger is effective in preventing motion sickness and settling an upset stomach. Take two capsules one hour before the trip and then one every couple of hours while traveling. For serious motion sickness, Cocculus homeopathic 30C every 4 hours is very helpful.

You can reduce jet lag when you are flying across time zones by staying well rested, drinking lots of water and adjusting to the new time zone by resetting your watch as soon as you are on the plane. Taking some extra Vitamin C and an immune booster like Echinacea will help increase the effectiveness of your immune system. When it is your new zone's time to wake up drink a strong dose of caffeine such as black tea or coffee. This is especially effective if you have not had any caffeine for several weeks. Spend as much time as possible in the sun, especially the first few days, to encourage your hormone systems to adjust to the new time.

The risk of a stroke while flying and immediately after can be high for many people, so avoid anything like alcohol which is dehydrating. Drink lots of water, take vitamin C and be sure to take your prescribed blood-thinner medicines regularly. Moving around the cabin every few hours is a good idea to avoid blood pooling in your legs. If you are drinking lots of water, juices and teas then you'll probably have to walk to the bathrooms regularly!

Changes in food and water can sometimes cause diarrhea while traveling. A good prevention if you are traveling in an area known for water problems, is grapefruit seed extract, a few drops in a glass of water daily. It important to have it diluted in water. In many areas of the world you should avoid drinking local water, ice and anything washed in the local water but not cooked. Peel all fresh fruits and vegetables. If diarrhea and vomiting occur, homeopathic Arsenicum album 30C, two pellets taken every few hours will help your system return to normal faster.

For quick healing of sunburns and cuts, use Calendula tincture (one dropperful in ¼ cup water) and spray or gently apply to the sensitive skin.

Hypericum oil applied directly to the skin stops pain, is antimicrobial and helps it heal. On a trip a girl fell off her bike and scraped up her legs badly. I quickly applied Hypericum oil over the scrapes and dirt. She rapidly calmed down and when we later irrigated the scrapes with water it didn't bother her at all until we got to one that had no oil on it, then she went through the roof. So, I knew it had really helped. I also gave her a couple pellets of homeopathic Arnica 30c under the tongue.

Frequently people are more active while traveling, using new muscles plus sitting for long periods of time in cars and airplanes. This can cause a general soreness, bruises or sore muscles. Rub Arnica ointment onto your sore muscles and bruises. In addition, taking a couple of pellets of homeopathic Arnica 30C can relieve the overall swelling and soreness after a long flight.

Rescue Remedy will help calm you should a crisis arise while traveling or if flying makes you nervous. Take a dropperful in a glass of water, straight in the mouth, or add some to your water bottle. After a very frightening experience, it is soothing but not sedating. If that isn't enough, then a single dose of homeopathic Aconitum napellus 30C is very helpful to clear and calm you. Aconitum also is good when you get chilled and feel like you are suddenly getting ill. A dose or two will restore your health.

DENTAL WORK AND SURGERY HINTS

DENTISTRY

Our teeth are very important to our overall health. Keeping them clean and checked regularly is as important as going to your naturopathic physician regularly to check your body's health.

If you require dental work, natural medicine will help you to heal faster, reduce the pain and prevent infection. People having dental work have their mouth open for a long time, causing soreness in the muscles. For that and for tooth extractions, I find that patients do very well with homeopathic Arnica Montana 200C afterwards. It helps control pain, the bleeding and swelling, thereby speeding the healing.

For a tooth extraction, a black tea bag, like Lipton, dipped in hot water, squeezed almost dry and placed on the tooth hole, provides tannins to help shrink the tissues and encourage clotting and healing. It is like a little hot pack on the area. Let it stay until it cools down.

If someone is having lots of dental work, nutrition can play an important part in their healing. A poor diet sets the stage for slower healing and can affect other aspects of health as well. Making sure there are adequate calories, protein, good fats, vitamins and minerals in the foods they can eat while their teeth are being worked on is very important. If their nutrition is being severely impaired, then they may need to slow down on the dental work.

Teeth cleaning does not affect homeopathy, but drilling and major work can affect a constitutional homeopathic remedy. Don't delay the work – but be sure to talk to your homeopath or naturopath before you make an appointment.

For sore or torn gums or problems with infection, Calendula and Hypericum tinctures in water (one dropperful each to ¼ cup) is a wonderful mouth wash. It speeds the healing and it can stop the pain when you have tooth infection or nerve pain. Swish it around in your mouth three times a day or as needed for pain.

Aloe vera is another very helpful plant for the gums. The house plant, Aloe vera officinalis, can be used for a topical application. Cut a two-inch section from the plant and peel all the external green off the clear gel inside. Make sure to get all the green off – it can upset your stomach. The larger, plumper stems can be less bitter. Insert the clear gel piece into your mouth between your cheek and on your infected gum. Leave it as long as is possible for maximum healing of your gums.

SURGERY

For elective surgeries, there are some important homeopathic remedies to have on hand to reduce apprehension, nausea from anesthesia, pain, swelling, bruising and to speed healing. Different surgeries can involve a unique combination of symptoms, so consult with a naturopath. In general, most people respond well to homeopathic Phosphorus before surgery to reduce apprehension, reduce bleeding during surgery and to help with nausea and vomiting from the anesthesia after surgery. Immediately after surgery, most patients respond well to homeopathic Arnica montana. Arnica reduces the swelling, pain and bruising so the body can heal more effectively. I encourage patients to take it every couple of hours as needed using pain as their indicator. Plastic surgeons use it frequently and successfully for reducing the bruising after surgery.

Generally, the potencies required for treatment around a surgery is higher than what is available to consumers. I usually recommend a 200C of Phosphorus taken a day before and then immediately before surgery. It can be repeated right afterwards if there is nausea and vomiting. The Arnica works best at the 200C or 1M level repeated every 3 to 4 hours. If you don't have access to the higher potencies, take whatever potency of Arnica you have available and it will help. It just might need to be repeated more often.

The following are some examples of common symptoms after surgery and the homeopathic remedy that might help. Nerve pain that is sharp and burning will respond well to homeopathic Hypericum. Abdominal surgery can require homeopathic Bellis perennis, a close cousin of Arnica, but more specific for surgery of the abdominal cavity, such as laproscopy. Staphysagria, also can be very helpful for ongoing abdominal pain after surgery.

Frequently a constitutional homeopathic remedy will stop working with the stress of surgery, so you need to talk with your homeopath about repeating it after you have recovered.

Herbally, I recommend that patients take a blood cleansing and immune stimulating herb like Echinacea to help their blood clear out any debris and chemicals from the surgery and also to help keep them from catching the illnesses lurking around in a hospital.

WATER THERAPY

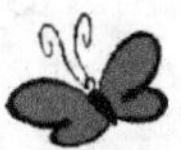

Old-fashioned hydrotherapy can provide a pleasurable boost to the body. Keeping your body warm is important for healthy circulation and a strong immune system. Alternating hot and cold will stimulate your immune system and improve positive blood flow throughout the body. Hot brings blood to the surface and cold pumps it back into the center. Creating a movement of the blood that helps the whole body. Pumping the blood at the feet, for example, also affects the head. Finishing with cold stimulates a positive rush of blood with lots of oxygen in it.

Various cultures have used hydrotherapy successfully over the ages. The Scandinavians use the sauna alternating with dips in snow or cold water. The Hawaiians used hot thermal pools and cooled in the ocean or light breeze. In my first sweat lodge, with a Navajo medicine woman, we came out of the sweat lodge between rounds from the intense steamy heat into a cool breeze and then returning to the sweat lodge. The secret is in the alternating of the hot and cold, to encourage the increase of oxygen and nutrients in the blood, therefore reducing congestion.

HOT FOOT BATH

Use a hot foot bath for bringing healing to foot issues, but also as a stimulant to the immune system for counteracting colds or flu.

Soak feet in hot water while wrapped in a warm wool blanket. Relax while you sit in a comfortable position for 10 minutes. Then dip feet in cold water and reheat the hot soaking water. Repeat hot and cold three times, ending with cold. Take care to avoid getting chilled after this treatment. Frequently this is used before putting on the warming socks and resting or sleeping.

WARMING SOCKS

After doing a hot foot bath, place a very well wrung out pair of wet thin, cotton socks on the feet. Cover with dry heavy wool (wool will pull the water away from the feet best) socks. Go straight to bed. When done properly, the socks will dry during the night. This increases the body's circulation and immune response. It can be used effectively during fever to help the body bring the fever down.

THROAT OR FACE THERAPY

Upper respiratory infections like sinusitis, colds and bronchitis respond well to alternating hot and cold water on the head and throat in the shower. I recommend doing it at least once a day when there is congestion in the head and throat. This works well when traveling since most homes and motels have a shower. It can help clear the head and sinuses for flying.

Take a shower and run hot water on the top of the head, face and neck. Then switch the temperature to run cold water, and again hot water. Alternate hot and cold at least three times and finish with cold water. This treatment increases circulation and increases white-blood cell activity and creates a lot of clearing and discharge from the sinuses.

One time my mother had to fly to a funeral just as she realized she was coming down with a head cold. By using alternating hot and cold-water therapy on her face and head before flying, in the motel and after the funeral, she was able to travel comfortably.

BEDTIME SINUS TREATMENT

Getting to sleep at night can be a big problem for people with sinus and lung congestion. Doing a steam delivers the herbs right to the surfaces where they are needed and helps with expectoration as well as calming. If someone is especially congested, they may need to do another steam in the middle of the night.

Bring a pot of water to a boil. Place a large mixing bowl on the table with a tablespoon of chamomile or lavender herbs in the bottom. You can also use a couple drops of essential oils, but I prefer the gentleness of the flowers. Pour boiling water in a bowl over the herbs. Sit at the table with a towel over both your head and the bowl to breathe in the steam and herbs for 10 to 15 minutes. You will have lots of drainage and be able to breathe easier afterwards because the herbs were able to get right where they are needed, in your lungs and sinuses.

SITZ BATH

This is used for urinary tract infections, prostate infections and to speed healing of the pelvic region. When you purchase the 40-quart plastic tubs – be sure that they are not too high and narrow, so you are able to sit in with your legs draped out.

What you will need:

2 tubs, 40-quart capacity each

Procedure:

- You need to be somewhat agile to do this safely or have an assistant to help you.
- Place one plastic tub into the bathtub and empty ice bags into it.
- Fill with cold water and slide to far end of the bathtub away from the water source.
- Place second plastic tub into bathtub and fill with hot water (as hot as tolerable)
- Stand in bathtub between the 2 plastic tubs.
- Gently sit into the hot water, with your legs hanging out. Turn immediately and sit into the cold water, legs always hanging out.
- Alternate between the 2 tubs, sitting longer and deeper (to about the level of your naval).

- Alternate until you are able to sit 2 minutes in hot and 2 minutes in cold.
- Repeat 2 minutes in hot, 2 minutes in cold at least 5 times.
- You may need to refresh the hot water.
- ALWAYS END WITH COLD WATER

CONSTITUTIONAL HYDROTHERAPY

Constitutional hydrotherapy is designed to bring the entire body and the immune system into balance. If you do not have a hot tub, sauna or steam room available there is still a way! This is one that is fairly easy to do at home.

SET UP: Place two large wool blankets on the bed. Cotton blankets do not work well because they get soggy. On top of the blankets place a cotton flannel sheet which you rinsed and spun in the washer machine. The washer machine is best because it will get the most water out without drying. Place a large dry towel at the head. Draw a hot bath.

PROCESS: Take a hot bath until you are very warm and sweating. When you come out your damp sheet will be cold from sitting in the air – this will be your cold aspect. Wrap yourself in the damp sheet and then wrap wool blankets around everything as an outer layer. Your head and neck should be wrapped in the towel and the blankets. It is best if the towel comes down over the eyes. Having someone available to help tuck you in tight is the very best. Your body will rapidly warm the damp sheet, your agitation will diminish and you will settle into a very calm and healing place. Plan on resting for at least 20 minutes.

EATING WELL AND FEELING WELL

Good nutrition includes enjoying what you eat as well as eating food healthy for your body. Hopefully you already enjoy the foods you eat, and they contribute to your good health, since your health reflects the food you eat. Eating is an essential activity that we all do several times everyday, so let's have fun with it! Eat what you enjoy; enjoy what you eat and be healthy.

REAL FOOD

Fresh fruits, fresh vegetables, nuts, beans, organic meats, clean oils and whole grains should be the staple of your diet. Eat as many organic products as you can, since this minimizes your exposure to pesticides, hormones and other toxins. I recommend following the conventional wisdom of at least five to ten servings of fruits and vegetables every day. This means having at least one fruit or vegetable serving for every meal in addition to fruit or vegetable snacks. Eating a mix of raw, steamed, frozen and canned can provide additional variety, eating a variety of fruits and vegetables each day.

Some easy ways I get more vegetables are through fresh guacamole, fresh salsas or spinach added to my breakfast eggs. For lunch adding onion, pickles, tomato and lettuce condiments on sandwiches and ordering sliced tomatoes and hot peppers on pizza increase the vegetable count. For several years when my daughters were young, we would count fruit and vegetable servings at dinner periodically to see how we were doing.

In addition, eating good quality oil is important for your whole body. Avoid artificial fats like the trans fatty acids in shortenings and margarines. I use extra virgin olive oil, organic coconut oil, organic butter and organic meats and dairy products. Supplementing the diet with Omega 3 fatty acids can dramatically improve health, helping increase brain clarity and reducing inflammation. Omega 3 fatty acids are found in high concentrations in fish oils, flaxseed and chia seeds. Seeds like sunflower and pumpkin or nuts like walnut, pecan and almonds provide wonderful oils as a complement. A snack of nuts and dried fruit keeps well, is tasty and is good for you.

When you look at protein, lean, organic meat is best. Eggs are rich in nutrients and protein and should be included in your diet. Foods such as beans, nuts and tofu are an important low fat and high fiber source of protein, but generally need to be combined for a complete protein.

One of the great benefits of eating whole, unpreserved foods is the increased fiber in the diet. Fiber is essential for the healthy functioning of the digestive tract and has been found to reduce the risk of many diseases. People that have not eaten many high-fiber foods in the past should increase their fiber-rich foods gradually to allow their body to adjust. Some examples of high-fiber foods are dried beans, dried fruits and the whole bran of grains. Grains like oats have a combination of soluble and insoluble fiber and both nourish the digestive tract plus provide bulk to prevent constipation.

A second advantage of eating fresh, whole foods is that you can relax knowing the micronutrients that are being discovered daily as suddenly "important" to good health are already in your diet. Our bodies have evolved over the centuries to perform optimally on whole, lean fresh foods and the ingredients in them. Science may never totally understand every vitamin, mineral and nutrient that is in food and important to good health, but our bodies know what to do with fresh, whole foods.

A third advantage in unpreserved and unprocessed foods is the energy they have to give us. Foods which have been minimally processed and would spoil if left out on the counter at room temperature still have active enzymes that assist us in their digestion. Our digestive system is a long fermentation unit and the only way foods get broken down is through enzymes and bacteria. That said, light steaming can be very helpful in breaking down the cellulose and improving the digestion of many vegetables. Beans and meats are better digested and safer after cooking.

ALL THINGS IN MODERATION

We have evolved as humans while eating a variety of foods. There is no single perfect food after we stop breast feeding. At six months of age even breast milk needs to be supplemented with food. A wide variety of foods yields the best nutrient base. I recommend not eating the same foods two days in a row. If you rotate basic ingredients like wheat, sugar and dairy every other day you will have less allergy problems.

Many of our packaged foods share similar ingredients that seem tasty but are not so good for our health: sugars, salt and hydrogenated fats. You may think you are getting variety, but actually you are eating the same thing in different shapes. For example, if sugar is the major ingredient in all the foods you are eating and drinking, then you are missing many important nutrients. Sugar may be called by a variety of names in the ingredient lists of foods: high fructose corn syrup, corn syrup, dextrose, fructose and sucrose are common labels. Soft drinks, fruit drinks and punch drinks are all primarily sugar. When something has only sugar and little or no nutrients, we call those empty calories.

Salt in moderation is important for many people. If you are working outside in the heat and sweating profusely, salt is essential to replace the sodium that gets lost in the sweat.

People with high blood pressure should discuss their salt intake with their health practitioner. Forty percent of Americans are salt-sensitive and sodium restriction may help lower their blood pressure. Many other factors, such as stress, contribute to high blood pressure. That includes stressors we have not yet identified.

MAINTAIN A HEALTHY WEIGHT

Eat when you are hungry and stop when you are full. It sounds simple but can be hard to practice. There are many and varied reasons for not following this simple rule. This is a key area where the mind-body connection is very visible. Listen to your body and eat only when you are hungry, not because you are thirsty, tired, stressed, or because your grandmother will be upset you didn't eat her dessert, or someone wants you to eat with them. Drink water if you are thirsty; rest if you are tired; and go for a walk, meditate or do Yoga if you are stressed. If you are not hungry you can always join a friend to enjoy the visit and eat lightly.

Learning to eat only when you are hungry starts right away with breast-fed babies. One of several benefits to breastfeeding is that the babies control how much they eat. They eat when they are hungry and stop when they are full. There is no external measure or monitor. Recently, new height and weight charts were released by the World Health Organization (WHO) for breast-fed babies. The WHO estimates that twenty percent of the world obesity is due to the many years using height and weight charts based on bottle-fed babies. Bottle-fed babies tend to be encouraged to finish the bottle, thereby overriding their sense of knowing when they are full. The new charts, based on a breast-fed baby's weight, suggests optimal weights that are twenty-five percent less than the old bottle-fed baby charts. Breast feeding has many other advantages, including enhanced bonding, a healthier immune system, increased intelligence and straighter teeth. I encourage families to make it a priority to breast feed their babies.

As we grow older, children and adults can maintain a healthy weight by eating at least three small meals a day and balancing their food intake between carbohydrates, proteins and fats at each meal. Regular physical activity is also key to maintaining a healthy weight. People eating a first meal, a break-fast including protein and do their exercising in the morning seem to speed up their metabolism, have more energy and are leaner. Balancing your food intake between carbohydrates, proteins and fats also means that your meals sustain you better. There aren't the blood-sugar peaks and valleys causing unexpected mood swings.

Eating regular meals also helps people to eat in moderation. Don't be afraid of fasting for 13 to 16 hours over night. This can be a reset to your system and appears to provide some health benefits.

Eat slowly and with small enough bites that you can chew the food thoroughly. The first stage of digestion is chewing and there is no other part of the digestive tract that can break up the food into small pieces as effectively. Once food is past the mouth it can only be broken down by acid, bacteria or enzymes. It takes about 20 minutes for your body to tell you it is full, so if you are chewing thoroughly and eating slowly, you will know when you are satisfied.

Drinking plenty of good quality, clean water can be very helpful to the proper functioning of the body. The body is about three quarters water and when you are low on water, you are dehydrated. Enzymes work better, elimination goes better, and the skin looks less wrinkly when the body has plenty of water. Very cold, iced drinks with meals which can inhibit proper digestion. Drinking tap water with its chlorine, fluoride and other toxic minerals can also be problematic. Chlorine and fluorine are a couple of the most toxic substances to life. Drinking spring water between meals is optimal. Most people find that 36 to 48 ounces of water a day keeps them hydrated.

Caffeine in excess creates problems with the adrenals and the breasts particularly. Adrenal fatigue can occur more readily when someone is drinking caffeine to keep going when they otherwise would be too tired. Your adrenals produce adrenalin, epinephrine, norepinephrine, cortisol, DHEA, testosterone, estrogen and progesterone. Coffee is a powerful herb that enhances creativity, but when abused over long periods of time overrides the body's feedback systems and can create health problems. Many women find that menstrual breast tenderness, ovarian cysts and other health concerns improve from stopping caffeine and coffee.

Nutrients that feed the adrenals are the B-vitamins, especially Pantothenic acid and Vitamin C. Taking supplements with these in them or eating lots of fresh fruits and vegetables is good.

SUPPLEMENTS

Regularly taking supplements like vitamins, minerals, antioxidants, herbs and other products from the health food store has become routine for many people. I see people with supplements ranging from nothing to large shopping bags full. One patient had so many supplements, they filled her car trunk and I had to go out to see them in the parking lot. As their number of pills increase, people wonder what is essential and what is not. There are many books written advising people on which supplements they should take, so I will give you my basic recommendations. Healthy people generally benefit from a capsule vitamin and mineral combination plus a sublingual B12 and some good flax or fish oils every day. In addition, they take Vitamin C along with immune stimulating herbs, such as Echinacea, when they feel run down.

Multivitamins and minerals have several hurdles to overcome from the bottle to your blood stream. The first big hurdle is you have to remember to take them. Next, they must have the ingredients you need in an appropriate balance. You must be able to dissolve them in your digestive tract. Last, you have to be able to absorb and utilize whatever form of the vitamin or mineral they are in. For all these reasons I encourage people to take supplements that are easy for them to remember, generally in capsules or liquid form plus inspected and certified to contain what is listed on the label.

A supplement that has been in the news a lot recently is Vitamin D. It is made in the skin from cholesterol and the sun. It is very helpful with a range of health issues, such as the bones, nerves and the immune system. The newest recommendations are at least 800 IU for people who are in the sun 15 minutes every day. Someone not getting much sun or with dark skin should be taking closer to 4000 IU especially in the winter.

Many of the essential minerals are not in adequate supply in our soils or foods. Boron, Selenium, Iodine, Zinc, Calcium and Magnesium are some we know are beneficial and should supplement regularly. Iron is essential for making blood and is very well conserved in the body. Too much Iron is toxic. Iron should not be taken as a supplement unless there is blood loss such as in menstruating women or demonstrated anemia from testing. Minerals especially seem to be hard to absorb from a tablet.   Over compression can occur in manufacturing, so I especially recommend a liquid or capsule as the best form to take minerals.

The B vitamins have been recognized for a long time as essential to health for all ages. Our adrenals, nervous system, skin and blood especially utilize the B vitamins for health. Pyridoxine, Vitamin B6, is the only B vitamin known to cause problems in high doses. I recommend that nobody take multiple doses of B6 and limit it to the recommended daily allowance per day. Folic acid and Vitamin B12 are best utilized in the body if they are taken as methyl folate (Folic acid) and methylcobalamin (Vitamin B12).   This is the form the body utilizes, so it does not have to convert them. In addition, Vitamin B12 taken under the tongue, or sublingual, is the most effective way to be sure it is going to be absorbed. If taken too late in the day B vitamins can disturb people's sleep, so I recommend that they not be taken after dinner time.   I see yellow urine as a good sign indicating the B vitamins have made it through the digestive tract into the blood and the excess is in the urine.

The fat-soluble vitamins such as Vitamin A and Vitamin E stay in the body, so large quantities should only be used with medical supervision. The precursor to Vitamin A is carotene and it is not a problem in large quantities, but again some people do not convert carotene to Vitamin A very well and so taking Vitamin A can be very helpful. Antioxidants such as CoQ10 can help the body retain it's Vitamin E and will strengthen the body's ability to deal with inflammation. CoQ10 also supports heart health.

Supplementing vitamins and minerals can be very beneficial to ensure adequate vitamins and mineral intake. However, it never replaces eating well as the best medicine. The synergy of eating well and taking appropriate supplements is where optimal health will arise.

Terminology

Acute illness or situation—having severe symptoms in a short course of time; i.e. colds, flu, etc.

Antidote—something that stops or neutralizes the healing action of a homeopathic remedy.

Case—as in "taking your case"; the process of questioning to determine the mental and emotional states and the physical symptoms of the patient.

Chronic illness—illness persisting for a long time; i.e. arthritis, allergies, diabetes, etc.

Classical Homeopathy—homeopathic medicine which is derived from and follows the teachings of Samuel Hahnemann, the founder of homeopathy. Only one remedy at a time is given under this system.

Constitutional—a remedy (or series of remedies) which affects the whole of the body and person. Used for curing chronic cases.

Expectorant—a substance that encourages the body's natural tendency to bring up phlegm, mucous, etc. from the respiratory tract.

Homeopathy—a system of medicine uses symptoms as a guide to increase the vital force. Based on the principle: "like cures like".

Immunoglobulins (Ig)—IgA, IgE and IgG are different forms of antibodies the immune system produces as protection, but which can cause allergic reactions if out of balance

Potency—the strength of the remedy based on the number of dilutions and potentizations of the mother tincture. Common potencies in the U.S. are 6C, 12C, 30C and 200C. The higher the number, the stronger the remedy.

Remedy—an energized dilution, derived from plant, animal and mineral sources. Available in many different potencies, the remedy is most commonly in pellet or water taken under the tongue.

Shopping List

ESSENTIAL MEDICINES TO HAVE ON HAND

Buy these items now as a beginning of your new first-aid kit.

- Arnica montana cream or ointment
- Calendula officinalis (Pot Marigold) tincture or cream
- Skin cream or ointment with Chaparral (Larrea tridentata) and Calendula
- Echinacea (Purple Coneflower) tincture
- Hypericum (St. John's Wort) tincture and oil
- Rescue Remedy – liquid, spray or pastilles
- Herbal sting-stop ointment
- Herbal teas
  Chamomile
  Lavender
  Licorice root
  Nettles
  Peppermint

ITEMS TO HAVE IN THE HOUSE
These are handy items to have in the house, available at most Grocery stores:
- Fresh onion
- Fresh garlic cloves
- Olive oil
- Fresh or dry parsley
- Vitamin C (as mineral ascorbate)
- Castor oil
- Witch hazel
- Epsom salts
- Hot Water bottle

Professional Organizations

American Association of Naturopathic
Physicians
4435 Wisconsin Avenue, NW, Suite 403
Washington, DC 20016
Ph. (202) 237-8150
www.naturopathic.org

National Center for Homeopathy
801 North Fairfax Street
Suite 306
Alexandria, VA 22314
Ph. (703) 548-7790
nationalcenterforhomeopathy.org

Council for Homeopathic Certification
PO Box 73
Lewisville, AR 71845
Ph. (866) 424-3399
www.homeopathicdirectory.com

MORE ON HOMEOPATHY

Homeopathy is a marvelous therapy for helping the body heal itself. When you cut yourself, isn't it amazing how the body knows just what to do to heal the wound? When the body does a good job of healing, it stays healed. We use homeopathy to bring the body back to balance, where it can do it's best healing.

Homeopathic remedies, or medicines, work differently from herbs and drugs because dosing is based more on when the body needs another boost. There is not the same chemical build-up in the body required like herbs and drugs. Our cells communicate in three ways we know of: chemical, electrical and color. Drugs and herbs use the chemical pathways, homeopathy uses the electrical channels, and color therapy is just now being explored.

Homeopathy has been around for two or three hundred years. Dr. Samuel Hahnemann spent a great deal of his life testing and writing about it. The beauty of homeopathy is that it stimulates the body to heal gently and effectively while doing no harm. However, you need the right homeopathic medicine for it to work. If a medicine does not work, then it is the wrong remedy, not the failure of homeopathy.

Homeopathy is a very individualized medicine. The challenge for people prescribing homeopathic remedies is to both understand the person's symptoms clearly and to know the remedies well enough to match them appropriately. The recommendations in this book are for acute situations where most people have similar symptoms, and these are the medicines most likely to help. If it does help, problem solved. If not, then another medicine needs to be selected.

Homeopathic potencies start in the stores at 6C and go up to 30C. Occasionally you can find Arnica in a 200C in the stores. The higher potencies are usually by prescription to avoid problems. People who don't understand remedies and repeat the wrong one excessively can create proving symptoms. The rule I recommend is to not repeat a remedy more than 3 times unless it is clearly helping. If it is relieving the symptoms, then continue to take as needed at the first return of symptoms. People who are used to avoiding conventional medicines as much as possible, will sometimes wait longer than needed, but their increased pain can interfere with healing. If a remedy is helping but has to be repeated very frequently, then a higher potency is needed.

A brief Materia Medica for the homeopathic remedies recommended in the book and in the accompanying kit is included. The remedy works best if it fits the individual being treated as closely as possible.

The National Center for Homeopathy is a wonderful source of information. Their magazine, <u>Homeopathy Today</u> is written with the consumer in mind. See their listing in References, Professional Organizations.

MATERIA MEDICA

Aconite (Aconitum napellus)- Used at the sudden onset of fever, shock or illness. After a terrifying experience it is very calming. It also works well for beginning flu or cold symptoms especially after getting chilled from dry cold wind or symptoms coming on at midnight. It is usually the first remedy to try with croup which comes on after midnight. Panicky or anxiety reaction with the fear of dying. Post traumatic stress treatment.

Apis mellifica – Allergic reaction, swelling, redness, insect stings where red and hot and swollen around the bite. Hives, edema, burning and stinging pain. Symptoms are worse heat and better cold and the patient is not thirsty.

Arnica montana – Post accident or trauma with shock, bruising, injuries, sprains or broken bones. The injured person says "I am fine and don't need a doctor" when they are obviously injured. Very sensitive to pain. Restless and cannot find a comfortable position. After a hard workout it will prevent sore muscles from overexertion. Useful before and after surgery and dental work to relieve discomfort and speed healing.

Arsenicum album – Food poisoning with diarrhea and vomiting, chilly, fearful, restless. A fear of dying. Craves cold drinks. Burning pain better with hot applications. Worse cold. Better warm drinks, warm weather and warm applications. This remedy is often very helpful for relieving the restlessness of dying animals or people, to ease their passing. A person needing this remedy can move constantly until exhausted. Thirsty for small sips of water.

Belladonna – Sudden, intense, throbbing pain. Redness and heat are frequently observed. The face can be red and eyes dilated. Early stages of an inflammation which comes on fast and intense.

Cantharis – Burning pains from sunburn, bladder infections or any first degree burn. Pain can be very intense. Pain on urination, constant urge to urinate.

Cocculus – Great travel remedy for motion sickness, effects of loss of sleep whether traveling or nursing the sick. Ailments from traveling.

Euphrasia – Watery eyes with hot or acrid discharge but bland nasal discharge. Allergies, conjunctivitis or colds with these symptoms.

Ferrum Phosphoricum – Early stages of acute illness and inflammations – fever with no other symptoms. Face alternates between red and pale. The first remedy many people take to clear the first sensation of cold or flu symptoms. Can joke and chat as though they aren't ill, just tired and with fever.

Hepar sulphuris calcareum – Abscess with chills. Very sensitive to cold drafts, pain, touch or smells and irritable. Sweats easily. Sticking, splintering pains. Yellow discharge. Colds, flu, coughs with these intense symptoms.

Hypericum perforatum – Injury to nerve-rich parts like fingers, toes, nose, lips and tailbone. Injury to brain and spinal cord. Violent shooting pains. Phantom limb pain. (we also use as herbal oil or tincture)

Kali bichromium - Sinusitis with ropy, stringy discharges of mucus. Intense pain in a single spot that can come and go suddenly or wander. Upper respiratory infections with thick, gelatinous discharges.

Ledum palustre - Puncture wounds, bites or stings with purpling and cold to the touch around the wound. Feels better with cold applications like ice packs, yet chilly overall and worse with warmth. Purple, swollen bruises or eye injuries.

Phosphorus – Nosebleeds or other bleeding of bright red, copious blood. Vomiting after anesthesia and surgery. Anxious, impressionable and sympathetic person, easily reassured. Electrical injuries and lightening strikes. Easily dehydrated. Desire for cold drinks, but may vomit them when they warm in the stomach.

Pulsatilla – Colds or flu with thick bland yellow to green discharges and a weepy feeling. Desiring consolation. Chilly, not thirsty, yet dry mouth. Better walking in open air. Changeable symptoms. Seen frequently with ear infections, colds, and bladder infections.

Rhus toxicodendron – Rusty gate feeling of joints – worse first motion, better continued movement and heat. Restless. After sprains and strains. Allergic skin reactions like poison oak/ivy.

Sarsaparilla – Bladder infection/cystitis for painful urination that is worse at the end of urination.

Silicea – Opens and clears abscesses. Expels foreign bodies imbedded in a person. For symptoms after vaccination. Chilly person, better with warmth. Chilly hands and feet. Easily tired

and easily chilled. Don't take repeatedly if have
any implants such as pacemakers.

Spongia tosta – Croup, asthma, bronchitis.
Croup is worse before midnight (Aconite at or
after) Cough is dry, like a seal's bark. Anxiety,
going to die from suffocation. Tickling and
dryness in throat. Frosty weather can help
cough.

Urtica urens – Hives, first and second degree
burns, insect bites. Stinging, burning pain with
scalding sensation. Genital burns. Serious
sunburns with burning and itching. Increases
milk production in nursing mothers.

Dr. Valeria Breiten

Dr. Valeria Breiten is a licensed Naturopathic Physician, Certified Classical Homeopath and Registered Dietitian. Her passion is teaching people to be healthier in a natural and sustainable way.

She received her B.S. from California Polytechnic State University, San Luis Obispo, California. Her dietetic internship was in Portland, Oregon. Dr. Breiten graduated from Southwest College of Naturopathic Medicine in Tempe, Arizona.

For more information visit her website www.DrValeria.net.